snowflake*

*Breaking Through Mental Health Stereotypes and Stigma

lucy nichol

WELBECK
BALANCE

Published in 2023 by Welbeck Balance
An imprint of Welbeck Trigger Ltd
Part of Welbeck Publishing Group
Based in London and Sydney
www.welbeckpublishing.com

A CIP catalogue record for this book is available from the British Library.

ISBN
Trade Paperback – 978-1-80129-217-7

Typeset by Lapiz Digital Services
Printed in Great Britain by CPI Group (UK) Ltd, Croydon CRO 4YY

10 9 8 7 6 5 4 3 2 1

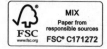

Note/Disclaimer
Welbeck Balance encourages diversity and different viewpoints.
However, all views, thoughts, and opinions expressed in this book are the
author's own and are not necessarily representative of Welbeck Publishing Group as
an organization. All material in this book is set out in good faith for general guidance;
Welbeck Publishing Group makes no representations or warranties of any kind, express or
implied, with respect to the accuracy, completeness, suitability or currency of the contents
of this book, and specifically disclaims, to the extent permitted by law, any implied
warranties of merchantability or fitness for a particular purpose and any injury, illness,
damage, death, liability or loss incurred, directly or indirectly from the use or application
of any of the information contained in this book. This book is not intended to replace
expert medical or psychiatric advice. It is intended for informational purposes only and
for your own personal use and guidance. It is not intended to diagnose, treat or
act as a substitute for professional medical advice. The author and the publisher
are not medical practitioners nor counsellors, and professional advice should be
sought before embarking on any health-related programme.

Every reasonable effort has been made to trace copyright holders of material
produced in this book, but if any have been inadvertently overlooked the publishers
would be glad to hear from them.

about the author

Lucy Nichol is a writer with a passion for mental health awareness. She has written extensively in the media, her words appearing in the *Independent*, the *i Paper*, *NME*, *Metro*, *Huff Post* and many more. She is also a former columnist with Sarah Millican's *Standard Issue* magazine, and has worked with a wide range of mental health charities including: Recovery Connections, Mind, Time to Change, Student Minds, Action on Postpartum Psychosis, Road to Recovery Trust, St Andrew's Healthcare and Newcastle United Foundation.

In 2021 she released her first novel, *The Twenty Seven Club*, a fictional and humorous exploration of mental health stigma and impact in the 1990s. Its sequel, *Parklife*, was released in 2022, focusing on the topic of addiction and recovery. She also had a short essay on anxiety published in Jonny Benjamin and Britt Pflüger's 2021 book, *The Book of Hope* (Bluebird).

She is, unfortunately, a bit of an expert when it comes to living with anxiety, and speaks openly about growing up with panic attacks and health anxiety. Lucy has also worked on behalf of several charities providing script advice for TV soaps and dramas regarding mental health (including addiction) portrayals.

For anyone who's ever been called a 'whiny needy twerp'
or an 'attention-seeking bastard' for speaking out about
a mental health problem

foreword

It is 2022 and sadly stigma is still alive and unwell in the UK, and in almost every culture across the globe.

We have made great strides over the last two decades to start to improve public attitudes and, more importantly, behaviour toward those of us who experience mental health issues … but lifting the burden of generations of prejudice and discrimination is no small task and neither is it a short-term pursuit.

There are many threats that can unravel these moves toward more progressive and just societies and the shifting of social norms.

Economic down-turns pose a risk to this progress as do negative high-profile mental health stories/events that secure wall-to-wall media coverage and trend on social media, with the reporting and social media chatter often reinforcing negative myths about dangerousness.

Social progress is also hostage to the fortunes of key opinion formers who dislike any form of moderation that threatens their right to air their views – views that often only serve to fuel stigma and discrimination that hampers millions of people's lives and, at the most extreme, puts lives at risk as people avoid or delay help-seeking due to shame and stigma.

This is where the "Snowflake" brigade march in …

Every 40 seconds someone in the world takes their life – mental health stigma (expressed externally from family, friends, managers, colleagues, teammates, fellow students and pupils, and the media) and internalized or self-stigma play significant roles in preventing early disclosure and help-seeking. Discrimination prevents us realizing our basic human rights – to a lover, partner, family, social life, work and income, and education.

When Care in the Community was the policy driver in the UK, I witnessed a huge vile and powerful backlash against it and, subsequently, the transformation of mental health provision in the 1990s. Sadly, the media, commentators and communities in general were not prepared for the housing of day services or supported accommodation on their streets or in their neighbourhoods (next door to their children's schools) and they were worried about house prices. I've kept many of those headlines and comments from media and social commentators, some from the mental health field itself, who said Care in the Community was a "social experiment gone horribly wrong and the Government have blood on their hands".

Sadly, what happened here in the UK is still is happening elsewhere in the world too – mental health policies and services change, but the public are not prepared for these changes; there is no mental health education at school, at home, at work or in the communities where people are going to be recovering and living.

Myths and misunderstanding are still prevalent in so many cultures with a very narrow view of the whole spectrum of mental health focused on crisis and an assumption that everyone with a mental health problem poses a danger to others. There is just no concept that there are millions and millions of us who do have a mental health problem working, parenting, governing, caring, and contributing to society in each and every village, town and city around the world.

COVID has pummelled the mental health and wellbeing of all our nations, with children and young people taking the brunt of this "mental health pandemic" – as I heard it described by mental health leaders at a recent global mental health summit.

Managing mental health issues was a central and core part of life for many millions of us before the pandemic – it is now a part of life for many more who have experienced mental health issues and psychological distress for the first time during this global pandemic, leaving a mental health legacy that will need attention for years to come.

The world seems to have woken up to mental health being an everyday issue for all of our populations, but I find it very sad that it seems to have taken a pandemic for us all to have come to the realization that mental health is just a part of being human, and we should treat it with the same respect as we do the rest of our health and wellbeing.

Can we really afford to entertain the views and offensive baiting of some social commentators who would rather put their own careers and financial gain ahead of the needs of our populations? Can we engage in more conversations about mental health and wellbeing, leading to more support from those around us, instead of being told to "man up" and stop being part of this "Snowflake Generation"?

If being a Snowflake means I talk more about what is bothering me, reach out for help, do things to take care of myself and others, and don't bulldoze my way through life causing harm and destruction in my path – then a Snowflake I am – and a proud one at that.

Stigma is still winning – but this book untangles its roots and shows us what we can do to change things.

As Edwin Mutura, one of the Campaign Champions I had the honour of working with in Kenya as part of the Time to Change Global Programme, says: "If I keep silent, stigma wins."

Sue Baker OBE
International Mental Health Consultant
Changing Minds Globally

contents

introduction

---

why i wrote this book

I never knew what panic attacks were when my first one decided to unleash itself from hell and knock me sideways. I was probably wearing a long dress with baseball boots. I had probably just eaten a cheese 'n' onion patty with chips and batter from Newland chippy. I was definitely a vegetarian – much to my parents' dismay. And I probably had a Rimmel Black Cherry lipstick, a single crushed-up Embassy No 1 and a few coins in my coat pocket that didn't add up to much. There definitely wasn't a mobile phone because I ran to the payphone to call my mum. Mobile phones didn't really exist then. At least, they weren't a reality for a 15-year-old girl from the north of England, anyway.

Mental health wasn't discussed then either, at least, not in a way that described what it really is. Instead, we talked about mad, crazy, scary "psychos". We watched horror movies featuring asylums and mental patients. We fell in love with the idea of the tortured rock star, and felt both enamoured and ridiculously out of our depth with our infatuations.

And we experienced mental health problems without knowing. Well, we *knew* but, more often than not, we didn't really know what it was that was wrong. We didn't know that we might in fact need therapy rather than iron tablets for those sick, frightening, faint spells. Of course, it was different for everyone, but I imagine that, even if you were diagnosed with a mental health problem back in the 1990s, you probably didn't tell many people for fear of being labelled crazy or weak or violent.

Today, the conversation has moved on significantly but, despite huge efforts by charity campaigns, ambassadors and activists, stigma still oozes like ectoplasm from dark corners and falls onto large crowds in wide open spaces like acid rain. Whether it's how someone might discreetly behave, choosing to drop a friend who has, for example, been admitted to a psychiatric hospital, or whether it's a troll on Twitter shouting "snowflake" or "wuss" or "just take a walk and get over it" at somebody struggling with depression – it still very much exists.

Stigma is a societal sickness that can cause distress and inhibit recovery and, put simply, it needs putting in its place – preferably in a locked box in a darkened room.

about snowflake

I've written this book to challenge the stereotypes we still hear to this day relating to mental health problems. Chapter by chapter I will break each stereotype down, discuss and debate why and how it is so wildly inaccurate.

- We need to understand what depression is … and what it isn't (i.e. feeling a bit sad).

- We need to understand what schizophrenia is ... and what it isn't (i.e. it isn't a split personality or a violent psychopathic trait).
- We need to understand what Obsessive Compulsive Disorder (OCD) is ... and what it isn't (i.e. it isn't a desire to arrange your bookshelves in a colour-co-ordinated fashion for Instagrammable purposes).
- We need to uncover and understand the stigma that still remains.

There are two key reasons why mental health stigma is important to me – and why it's something I am so keen to challenge.

Firstly, as already mentioned, as a teen, I developed an anxiety disorder that manifested as panic attacks and extreme health anxiety. If anyone spotted me, age 15, on my knees, retching, dizzy and hanging onto the railings on a busy street, in the middle of my first ever panic attack, they might have pointed at me and said, "What the hell is that nutter doing?". If I had heard that, I would have felt really ashamed. I might have been too embarrassed to see the doctor or the counsellor I was subsequently referred to. And my anxiety might have got much, much worse with no treatment or therapeutic outlet. Luckily, I never heard such comments. But I'm not suggesting that any person saying that would have *meant* me harm. They might have been unnerved by me. I certainly was!

I'm therefore categorically not suggesting that anyone who inadvertently uses mental health stereotypes or stigma should endure a Twitter pile-on or an equally horrific ghosting/cancelling.

Secondly, I have experienced stigma and discrimination in the workplace. A few years ago I went to see the doctor as my panic attacks had made an unwelcome return. I was convinced the bus was going to topple over and smash us all to smithereens below the flyover, and that my throat was going to randomly choke me. Around the same time, work became incredibly stressful. I never knew how my anxiety was going to manifest. Was I going to be shaking in a corner like Cringer from *He-Man*, or was I going to become as uncompromisingly angry and raging as the Incredible Hulk? Perhaps, as was more common, I would sit on my panic attacks trying desperately to suffocate them and keep them hidden from open-plan-office eyes. That is, until I no longer could ...

Unfortunately, these moods that I felt unable to do much about soon became part of my annual review at work, depicted by a big squiggly line drawn on a piece of paper. I couldn't argue with it, but I also wanted to scream about how unfair it was. I wasn't enjoying my moods, I wasn't on some kind of high. Inside, I felt desperate, preoccupied with whether or not my food would choke me and whether or not I'd need to get off the bus a few stops early on the way home again.

And I've also experienced self-stigma – being unable to share my experiences with my friends when I was growing up in the 1990s. I didn't really understand them and I felt quite ashamed. Anyone with a mental health problem will know how exhausting it is trying to sit on said mental health problem and keep it quietly hidden, when inside your brain and body you're actually experiencing a panic attack. You *could* say it's like trying to hold in a fart in a public place – forever!

Being able to simply say to someone, "I think I'm having a panic attack," usually, in my experience anyway, limits the amount of time the panic lasts. Because telling someone and not having to pretend is like turning on a tap. You're gradually releasing a little bit of the pressure (or gas – if we're sticking with the fart metaphor).

But when it comes to the person who drew that dramatic wiggly line in my annual review, and the person who suggested I didn't have anything to be anxious about, I am not angry with them. I just wish I had been able to calmly articulate why they were wrong to say such things at the time. Instead, I felt ashamed, angry, frustrated and stupid. And those feelings can make your mental health even more challenging.

Was the person who drew the squiggly line wrong to do so? I mean, it was kind of accurate. However, as I have come to believe, they *were* wrong to raise this in the context of my annual review.

I didn't really know much about stigma at the time. I'd seen the Mind and Time to Change campaigns, but I thought they were more about raising awareness. I didn't understand that they were actually about raising awareness *responsibly*.

I want this book to encourage us all, through words and ideas, through expert comment, and through crowd-sourced comment and observations, to consider how language can affect people and to be more mindful about how we use our words when it comes to conversations about mental health. In writing this, I too am still learning.

what this book is ... and what it isn't

This is categorically *not* a book of rules. It will not tell you what you can and can't say to someone with a mental health problem – or to anyone for that matter. It won't lay into people who have inadvertently used stigmas or stereotypes, not least because *I'm* guilty of that myself. As a child growing up in the 1990s, I used to talk about the "nuthouse" down the road. I didn't understand mental health stigma as a kid, and I didn't know what someone with a mental health problem "looked like" (even though they were staring back at me in the mirror). Also, testament to this is the fact that this so-called "nut house" wasn't even a mental health hospital. It was supported accommodation for people with learning disabilities. We were completely and utterly wrong in our assumptions.

However, I'm not in therapy revisiting my youth and metaphorically kicking my younger self up the arse. I meant no harm. I was a child, after all, with a lot of learning to do. But I'm *so glad* I learned, because even though I *meant* no harm, it's quite possible I could have *caused* some harm.

context is key

I once wrote an article for *The Independent* on addiction stigma. It was really positively received aside from one point – I was called out for using the word "addict". At first, I felt pretty pissed off. I was trying to do something good, after all. My ego got a bit of a battering and I couldn't understand why there was such an outcry. I'd worked with 12-step recovery charities, where many people who had lived experience of addiction referred to themselves as "addicts". But that's where context comes in – it was their prerogative how they referred to themself and their own experiences.

As somebody writing on such a high-profile platform, people had every right to challenge me and my words. It was an opinion piece – I was putting it out there to provoke and affect change. It was open to critique and debate. That's the whole point of op-eds. So, in addition to facing up to what percentage of my upset was actually ego-driven, I decided to no longer talk of "addicts" but rather "people who have experienced addiction". Considering this when I write really doesn't affect me much or cause me any hassle. It's no big deal. But to someone who has experienced addiction or related problems, who might not embrace the label of "addict", my inability to change the way I write could cause upset or offence. Because nobody is just "an addict" – people are people. And understanding that is key to recovery.

I'm writing as someone who has experienced stigma, and as someone who wants to continue to learn because I've got it wrong many times myself – and I imagine I'll do so again some day. So, in each chapter, you'll find me and a range of mental health experts breaking down some of the more common mental health stereotypes.

contributors

I've been incredibly lucky to get to know and work with a bunch of truly awesome people, so in these pages you'll be able to soak up insight from lived and professional experiences from (in alphabetical order):

- Catharine Arnold – author and historian
- Sue Baker OBE – international mental health consultant
- Jonny Benjamin MBE – mental health campaigner and author
- Dr Helen Casey – psychologist
- Ruth Cooper-Dickson – positive psychology practitioner
- Richard Cunningham – Safer Communities Co-ordinator
- Natasha Devon MBE – mental health campaigner, radio presenter and author
- Amy Dresner – author of *My Fair Junkie*, journalist and former comedian
- Claire Eastham – mental health campaigner and author

- Adam Ficek – musician with Babyshambles and psychotherapist
- Dr Stephanie de Giorgio – GP
- Maureen Herman – writer and former musician with Babes in Toyland
- Dr Jess Heron – CEO, Action on Postpartum Psychosis
- Beverley Hunter – Research & Evaluation Communications Lead, Fulfilling Lives
- Dr Kelechukwu Ihemere – senior lecturer in Linguistics and English Language at the University of Westminster
- Shahroo Izadi – behavioural change specialist and author
- Cara Lisette – mental health nurse, eating disorder campaigner and author
- Dr Craig Malkin – Harvard psychology lecturer, psychologist and author
- Catrina McHugh MBE – Artistic Director, Open Clasp Theatre
- Dr Luna Muñoz Centifanti – psychologist
- Dot Smith – CEO, Recovery Connections
- Hope Virgo – mental health campaigner and author
- Bernie Wong – senior manager of insights and principal, Mind Share Partners

Together, we're going to explore some of the most persistent mental health stereotypes. From over-sensitive snowflakes to attention-seekers, and from psychos to winos and addicts, we're going to look at when, why and how these stereotypes are used in society, and why they are so completely and utterly wrong and, more importantly so, why that makes them so dangerous.

whopping big disclaimer

Please bear in mind when reading that people's views change over time and they can be affected by personal life experiences (rather than fads as some of this book's critics will no doubt suggest). It might be that something I say, or something one of the book's contributors says, might not resonate with you. And that's OK. We are not perfect and, anyway, the world would be boring if we all thought the exact same things, enjoyed the exact same movies and went for the same Krispy Kreme in the Krispy Kreme cabinet.* In fact, you might not even want to go in the Krispy Kreme cabinet at all. You might prefer crisps.

When people prefer crisps and decide to take out the entire Krispy Kreme cabinet anyway because they're the biggest, loudest or first in line, smashing the delightful doughnuts into one big squishy inedible mess, well, that's just a pointless waste of time. And pretty mean, actually.

It's the same when it comes to talking about mental health. It's about intention. But to the trolls who trample on somebody else's personal preference or experience, calling them a snowflake or an attention-seeker, when it literally has no bearing on said troll, I'll just say this: SHUT UP AND MOVE THE FUCK AWAY FROM THE DOUGHNUTS!

Just like it's actually really easy for *anyone* with good intentions to start a conversation about mental health (you don't need to be a neurologist or a psychologist to do that), it's easy *not* to fuck it up with a dangerous or controversial agenda. For most of us getting it wrong, it's often a slip-up, a trip, a lack of understanding as to why it's wrong to use such a stereotype – or even that it's a stereotype in the first place. Hence the reason this book exists: to give us more confidence in our own experiences, to support others through our conversations and to have a logically rounded, rational argument to use in response to shouty insults such as "Snowflake".

Happy reading …

(*I don't care whether or not this metaphor is ridiculously tenuous. I love Krispy Kremes.)

1

why language matters

When it comes to mental health, why is language so important? How can words alone help somebody recover from a mental health problem or, conversely, make somebody's mental ill health worse? Can words *really* have that much power? After all, they're only words, right?

But the thing is, if they're "only" words, why do our lives, literally, revolve around them? They tumble out of the mouths of heroes and villains, and they can be as powerful as spinach is to Popeye and as devastating as Kryptonite is to Superman. Words matter. If they didn't, we wouldn't be so hopelessly devoted to them.

In today's world, words have even more longevity. A spur-of-the-moment drunken tweet can resurface online many years later, and past sensationalist media stories can be the first things to pop up when someone's googling symptoms of a mental health condition. Imagine how such stories might make you feel when you're distressed or confused about something you're going through? Adding shame and stigma into the mix could stop you from opening up and seeking help.

Yesterday's news is no longer simply "old news" that's been confined to fish 'n' chip wrapping. Yesterday's news lingers online like a powerful stink bomb ready to unleash its toxicity whenever someone happens to stumble across it. Subsequent clicks and shares reignite the story, furthering its harmful reach and impact.

This is why we need to redress the balance. And this is why language matters.

I spoke to Dr Kelechukwu Ihemere, a senior lecturer in Linguistics and English Language at the University of Westminster, about the importance of words. Dr Ihemere provides an interesting angle on this. "While there is no denying the fact that the damage sticks and stones can cause can go deeper than the surface and result in emotional trauma and distress, we often recover from the physical damage over time. However, as words escape our mouths or fingertips through typing, it's very onerous to take them back and they have the capacity to create fortresses in people's minds that can tremendously limit their self-worth, dismantle their self-esteem or destroy them mentally. This negativity carries over to how these individuals view the world as closing in on them."

Dr Ihemere also talked about how the words we choose don't just convey literal meaning – they also have the capacity to convey our attitudes and beliefs about the way the world should work. They reflect our deeper thoughts and ideas.

Put simply, words can build – or destroy. They're a powerful tool that we are blessed with. And just as we should never underestimate the power of a politician's dodgy haircut in undermining the serious nature of his actions, neither should we underestimate the power of words in undermining an individual's self-esteem and crippling their mental wellbeing.

why and how does language change over time?

Dr Ihemere told me that you simply can't divorce language from our customs, traditions and overall culture and that, in fact, language is a culture purveyor. He said: "Those arguing that language should not offend maintain this argument up to the point where it is about the other. However, when it is an issue about *their* language and culture, then it matters, and they will raise hell to fight their corner."

Isn't that interesting? Funnily enough, when so-called "snowflakes" bring up the subject of words and language, they often provoke an equally intense response from the angry red-faced people who called them "snowflakes" in the first place. People on *both* sides of the argument have been made equally angry about the subject of language. Which proves the point that words mean a lot to *all* of us.

But why does language change over time anyway? And why has there been so much discussion around it in relation to mental health? Dr Ihemere said: "As we experience our world in new ways, old words come to acquire new meanings and erstwhile meaning can become narrower and more specific to the point that they might no longer be fit for current intents and purposes. Thus, an important component of being an effective communicator is being sensitive to gauge the effects of our word choices on the hearers and be able to make necessary adjustments."

During our conversation, Dr Ihemere brought up the case of a BBC Radio 1 DJ who was reprimanded for describing a particular song as "gay"– using this word to imply that the record was not very good. But using this word in that context is clearly unacceptable to those in society who are gay, as it infers that there is something wrong with them or that they are sub-human.

He said that our language evolves as we interact with speakers from different backgrounds in our contemporary, more diverse, communities. Therefore words that were acceptable to us decades ago fall out of favour as our communities change and grow. He added: "It therefore becomes necessary for us and our language to evolve to accommodate the present realities of multi-ethnic and multi-cultural communities."

responding to a changing society

From our time chatting, I started to really understand what it is that makes language so alive, fluid and energetic. As Dr Ihemere pointed out, it needs to flex as society changes, just as fashion and gesture do. Even law plays a part here ...

In conversations about mental health, for example, we have changed how we talk about suicide. The term "commit suicide" used to be a fairly accurate description because, up until 1961, suicide in England and Wales was indeed a crime. So, just as you might "commit theft" or "commit murder" you might also "commit suicide". More than *half a century* since the change in law, however, the term "commit suicide" is still used.

When you stop and think, it's a pretty horrendous thing to say of someone who took their own life, probably due to severe mental health difficulties. And if there's one thing that will surely stop you opening up to someone about suicidal thoughts, it will be the fear of being labelled a criminal on top of everything else you might be going through.

It's problematic because using the phrase "commit x" refers to a criminal act and implies that the person is doing something that makes them a bad person. Being suicidal doesn't make you a bad person – it makes you vulnerable and in need of care, support and empathy.

If you want to consider just how much things have changed since suicide stopped being a criminal act, then bear in mind that it was just one year earlier, in 1960, that Penguin had to fight an obscenity case following the publication of DH Lawrence's *Lady Chatterley's Lover*. And it was 1967, another six years *after* suicide was decriminalized, before gay sex was decriminalized for men over 21 years of age.

Society has moved on a lot, so it makes sense to challenge language hangovers from those relatively oppressive times doesn't it? It makes sense to suggest that we should consider removing the word "commit" and instead say "died by suicide" or "completed suicide" because it's no longer accurate. It's not about being finicky and over-sensitive – it's been a whopping 50+ years since the change. So it's hardly a radical change.

the case for nuance

Just like our mental health exists on a spectrum, the debate around language and sensitivity exists on a spectrum. At one end, you have those who know full well that they are inciting hate or causing harm by using stigma and yet continue to do so regardless. I'm talking mainly about trolls or those who have big media or social media platforms and use them to shame others – or others' experiences.

At the other end, you've got a similarly angry tone from those publicly berating every. single. individual. who happens to get it wrong through lack of knowledge or understanding.

Even if both extremes directed their angst exclusively toward each other, it still causes harm to those who are listening in to the conversation – those who are hearing that their mental health problem makes them "weak" or those who once said they were "depressed cos their team lost the match" and now feel they have committed a heinous crime (you *haven't* committed a heinous crime, but there's nowt wrong with exploring the effects of language and its impact and adapting how we communicate. I like to reflect and learn all the time. It's like maple syrup and porridge for the soul. Warm, sweet and wholesome).

Neither extreme on the spectrum is healthy. But I *do* think we should be able to embrace a changing society and therefore an evolving language. We are all human, and we all make mistakes. The key to being kind, I believe, is accepting when we might have made a mistake or caused offence – whether that be by using a stereotype or by overzealously challenging someone who meant no harm.

Nuance is all too often lost. We are not a bunch of tabloid headlines – we are people. And if we tweet something well-intentioned, but stigmatizing, we just need to have the courage to reflect on it and throw our hands up when we've got it wrong. It does, of course, take strength to do that, but the pay-off is always worth it.

Another point to consider is that, just because somebody has contributed to a story that has a negative or stigmatizing headline, it doesn't mean that their contribution is bad or wrong. Beyond the headline, we might discover an article that incorporates a real life, genuine case study and, regardless of what we believe the intentions of the journalist or editor to be, we can still empathize with the case studies *within* the article. We can be both angry at the author/editor *and* sympathetic to the interviewees.

There are far too many incidents where we become entirely polarized. But when was life ever black and white? I've been guilty of it – I'm sure most of us have at some point. But we need to debate and we need to challenge. We also need to be kinder when someone makes a genuine mistake. A patient and well-intentioned challenge could change hearts and minds. Quote-tweeting to shame someone publicly who, for example, says "I'm 'a bit OCD' because I like colour co-ordinating my bookshelves" isn't going to have a positive effect. What harm might we be doing to that person if we encourage an angry pile-on?

A genuinely kind and diplomatic approach, however, might just help us understand one another a bit better. After all, nuance is a thing we human beings should wholeheartedly embrace. Cos there aren't many mammals able to pull it off.

the impact of language on mental health

The reason language matters so much when it comes to mental health is because people react to words – and that doesn't just mean they get "upset" by them. People act on things that they hear and believe. If you confuse psychopathy and psychotic (more on that later), you might find yourself ditching a friend because you think they're akin to the murderous Villanelle in *Killing Eve* or a danger to your bunny rabbit or pet puppy (1980s' and 1990s' film references there).

If you confuse your co-worker who has OCD with "being a bit like Monica from *Friends*", you'll underestimate their reaction to your "harmless" little joke of emptying the waste-paper bin on their desk. This is because you've heard that people who are tidy are "so OCD" and not equated the acronym to the debilitating illness that so many people struggle to live with.

So, there's our understanding of the *definition* of words, phrases and medical terms that we need to consider in relation to mental health. But there's also inference and attitudes. If, for example, we dismiss depression because we don't fully understand it, the person experiencing it may feel that they really should "just get over it". Depression isn't a state of feeling "a bit down", it's not something you can "just snap out of". It's an illness. But if you feel ashamed about how your depression is making you feel and act, it will inhibit recovery. It might stop you asking for help, it might cause you to bottle things up when directing negative thoughts and beliefs toward yourself is clearly not conducive to recovery. Mental health problems can often thrive on negativity and isolation – whereas recovery thrives on care and support.

There are "Impact" sections in the remaining chapters featuring anonymous quotes from people who have been adversely affected by stigma and the language attached to it. They describe how it has made them feel or behave so we can see the reality of the impact our words.

The impact of stigmatizing words and language can leave a nasty imprint for a long, long time. So, it has to be worth our time debating the subject, listening to others and reflecting on our own use of words.

the case for change

We shouldn't fight for freedom of expression *only* when it suits us. If we *truly* believe in freedom of expression, then we should listen to others' views as well. I don't think it's about policing language or being over-sensitive, it's just about considering others and not holding onto something out of tradition or some misguided principle. Is saying "committed suicide" really that important to hang onto? Will it make your life any worse off if you changed how you referred to suicide?

Rather than "bowing down" to "snowflakes", is this perhaps more about a fear of change? A desire for the world to remain static? We all love a bit of nostalgia, but as much as I'm obsessed with 1990s' music and the recipe that Sainsbury's used to make their frozen cheese and tomato pizza circa 1991, I wouldn't want to give up my iPhone or Netflix in exchange for them. We need to adapt, consider and flex to create a world in which everyone can feel comfortable and respected. A world in which we can embrace new opportunities and reflect fondly on positive moments in our history. It's about balance – it's not about simply having it one way or another.

British comedian Russell Brand is a great example here. Have you ever come across any other man who uses the English language in all its wondrous traditional glory, and yet manages to perfectly intertwine it with a gazillion fucks and the occasional gritty tale of heroin addiction? In 2014, according to a piece by *Guardian* journalist Laura Barton,

Russell Brand's testimony to a parliamentary committee (along with writer Caitlin Moran's tweets) were to be studied as part of the A-Level English Language syllabus. The article reports on the outrage that poured in after this was announced by the exam board.

So, clearly, it's not simply outrage about words being seemingly "stolen" by woke snowflakes that we're dealing with, but outrage about embracing the new, too. If we can ask ourselves why we are *genuinely* displeased about today's society recommending a change in how we talk about suicide or about a word disappearing from a song, we might find that our only real grievance is our own lack of understanding.

Let's dig a bit deeper before we get angry about any more lost or found words.

2

don't call me ... attention-seeking

There's going to be a fair bit of irony in this chapter. At least, I *think* there is and I hope I haven't misinterpreted the word like Alanis Morissette apparently did in the 1990s (we all forgive the mighty Ms Morissette, though, right?).

The irony I speak of comes in the form of individuals spewing out the term "attention-seeker" all over social media in reference to people who talk about their mental health problems or who are suicidal. The reason I find this ironic is because, in making such a fuss about so-called "attention-seekers" the authors of such posts are, undeniably, seeking attention.

"attention-seeking b*stards"

In 2015, HuffPost posted an article sharing several tweets written by commentator and business woman Katie Hopkins on the subject of mental ill health. One stated that being diagnosed with depression was "the ultimate passport to self-obsession" and another called suicidal people "attention-seeking b*stards".

We've seen similar tirades from TV presenters and journalists. For example, in 2017 Piers Morgan tweeted that Will Young "does not have PTSD, he has WNTS. Whiny needy twerp syndrome". This story ran in several newspapers and he was of course criticized by mental health campaigners.

But when it comes to talking about our own mental health problems, there are two key considerations. Firstly, it's helpful to others. To openly discuss things that are (clearly) still stigmatized helps others to feel less alone and less ashamed. It might encourage somebody to recognize their own symptoms or behaviours as something that can be treated or managed. They might see that there *is* a light at the end of the tunnel because, after all, here's somebody tweeting/blogging/vlogging, etc. who's also been to rock bottom and is now thriving.

Secondly, *we* might need some help or peer support ourselves. We might be lacking something specific from our friends or family – perhaps recognition of some of the symptoms we are experiencing – and therefore we seek interaction with others who truly get it. That's why there's a strong and supportive mental health community out there – we relate to each other. I've often put out a tweet when I've been struggling with an obsessive thought about my health or a panic attack trigger – and the response I've received has always helped me because it's come from others who have been there. It's invaluable.

attention-seeking ... to get a message out

My (unsurprising) view on celebrity ambassadors for mental health awareness is that they are trying to start conversations and show others that there is hope and they should not be ashamed of experiencing a mental health problem. Rather than seeking attention they are trying to show that mental illness doesn't discriminate, and that any of us could be affected at some point in our lives.

We need to remember that mental health campaigners and ambassadors are often, as a result of this work, dealing with a lot of difficult and worrying conversations that come their way, trying to navigate or signpost people to support and working with charities to ensure that the huge response that they see from their openness is carefully monitored – this also involves ensuring that *they* have the relevant support they need when hearing difficult or traumatic stories from others.

Being a mental health influencer, campaigner, activist or ambassador – whatever you want to call it – is not something that's simply just fun to do. It's not just a nice way of raising your profile. I have had to seek support from Time to Change and The Samaritans to deal with conversations on social media that made me concerned for an individual's safety; so, imagine if you had half a million plus followers, like many celebrities do. The bigger the impact (or attention) that comes as a result of a celebrity speaking out, the more time and resource they are required to put in to support the people they have reached.

The response to your work is not something that you can easily switch on and off, and charities who work with celebrity ambassadors do a lot to protect both the ambassador and the individuals who feel able to speak out as a result of raising awareness. It's a positive outcome, but it's certainly not easy-peasy!

is seeking attention actually a bad thing?

Let's look at what attention-seeking actually is – as it's so often downplayed as a frivolous or greedy action.

Perhaps sometimes attention-seeking *is* egotistical. Perhaps, in some instances, someone is topping up the huge amount of attention that they're used to and that they enjoy. But there are reasons why we shouldn't automatically view what we perceive to be attention-seeking as an egotistical frivolity. Perhaps we should consider why the person needs the attention. What's missing from their life?

I asked positive psychology practitioner and trauma-informed coach, Ruth Cooper-Dickson, her views on attention-seeking. She said: "There is actually a personality disorder – called histrionic personality disorder – that involves what we might call attention-seeking behaviours. In the DSM (*Diagnostic Statistical Manual*) it describes a pattern of excessive emotionality. In fact, the word histrionic is derived from a Latin word to mean 'actor' or 'player'. There are usually key symptoms or behaviours involved, including being uncomfortable in situations where he or she is not the centre of attention, inappropriate interactions with others that might be sexual or provocative, use of physical appearance to draw attention to self and self-dramatization. So there is certainly a personality disorder associated with this kind of behaviour but even then, it is a serious and incredibly challenging psychological state for anyone to be living with."

Ruth told me how sometimes this attention-seeking behaviour stems from childhood, where people haven't been recognized, affirmed or validated in the past. She explained how, in these cases, the behaviours can persist into adulthood and, when people are really struggling to ask for help, they might act out in different ways, often not really being conscious of how it comes across.

Ruth added: "So we have to consider, is it attention seeking or attention *needing* – is there a reason that somebody genuinely needs that attention?"

Mental health researcher and campaigner, Natasha Devon MBE, said something similar: "People seek attention because they *need* some attention. That really is the long and short of it. Unfortunately, what they often get is the wrong sort of attention and they're often not able to differentiate between that and the type of attention that would help them navigate whatever challenge they are facing."

And mental health nurse and campaigner, Cara Lisette, added: "Attention, in its various forms, is a basic human need. It is often looked down upon but, ultimately, if somebody is seeking attention, it means there is a need not being met somewhere – be that physical, emotional or social. Not all of us grow up learning the safest and more 'socially acceptable' ways of gaining the attention that we need, and many people who end up using maladaptive strategies to have their needs met have tried many different methods before resorting to ones that are harmful or frowned upon. There are many reasons why people might be trying to gain attention from others, and it's important to recognize that most of us are doing this in the most effective way we have learnt to, regardless of whether this may be considered healthy or not."

tackling the stigma

I'm starting to think that being an attention-seeker isn't really the issue; it's our *understanding* of what it means to seek – or need – attention in the first place that's the problem. The term itself is stigmatized.

What's wrong in saying, "I need something from you? I need someone to listen to me?" We should never be too quick to dismiss anyone as "just an attention-seeker" because they may genuinely be reaching out for help. Some people *might* constantly seek attention, but they may have a deep need for it. That's not a nice place to be. Surely, if we were just having a bit of fun, wanting the spotlight on us and having a jolly old time racking up likes or follows, wouldn't we be better off filming ourselves vogueing or moonwalking (to show my age a moment) and sticking that on TikTok?

Ruth added: "From a mental health first aid point of view, if anyone suggests that they are going to harm themselves by telling someone or posting it on social media, we always, *always* take those kinds of statements seriously. We always need to act on them. People *really* don't say these things for a laugh."

And as someone who visits hundreds of schools and colleges to talk about mental health, Natasha is often asked about self-harm and how we can tell the difference between self-harm for attention-seeking and self-harm when someone is genuinely distressed. She said: "There's so much wrong with that question. We should treat *all* self-harm seriously and remember that people experiencing mental health issues aren't always easy to sympathize with. In fact, like anyone, they can sometimes be really annoying. They're still in distress and they still need support, regardless."

a note on self-harm

A dangerous narrative has developed around self-harm being an attention-seeking behaviour or "trend". But this couldn't be further from the truth. So, there is clearly a huge misunderstanding around *why* people self-harm.

Firstly, self-harm is often done privately – behind closed doors. If it was simply an attention - seeking behaviour, surely that wouldn't be the case.

But there are also misconceptions around the *intended outcomes* of self-harm. For example, self-harm doesn't always coincide with suicidal thoughts – and this again feeds into the attention-seeking idea. When somebody has cut themselves, for example, I've seen people jump straight to the conclusion that the individual was trying to convey suicidal feelings without actually meaning to go through with it – which then, sadly, is all too often categorized as "just attention-seeking".

But it's far more complex than that. Cara said: "There are many reasons why people might harm themselves: it can be to feel physical pain, as a punishment, as a distraction, as a grounding technique, to try to change their appearance or to show distress without needing to verbalize it. Some people self-harm as a way to communicate they are hurting to others. Whatever the reason, self-harm always serves a purpose and meets a need, even if the individual themselves isn't always aware of what that is."

In addition to her professional experience of working with individuals who have self-harmed, Cara has personally struggled with it herself for many years. She said: "I was relatively secretive about it and it was very connected to my eating disorder; I used self-harm as a punishment when I wasn't able to follow the rules my anorexia dictated to me perfectly, or as a way of harming my body because I hated it."

It's easy to think of self-harm as being just one type of behaviour (e.g. cutting or burning) and yet there are actually many different ways in which we *all* self-harm from time to time. Just as our mental health can be good or bad without necessarily being diagnosable (i.e. we can be elated without being manic, or sad without being depressed), we might all self-harm occasionally without it having a particularly negative impact on our lives. As Ruth explained: "It's helpful to think of self-harm on a continuum. For example, we all have behaviours like smoking, drinking, online spending, eating too much, gambling at weekends, etc. that we turn to for some kind of relief. Risk-taking behaviours like these are all forms of self-harm.

"I have personally experienced using exercise and disordered eating practices to manage what was happening outside of my control. I was exhausting my body through exercise to stop myself feeling anything emotionally or mentally and just really pushing my body to its limit. But perhaps the reason we don't always think of these things as forms of self-harm is because we find them more acceptable."

Natasha agrees. She said: "We can think of self-harm according to two defining factors. The first is that it is something which we know, logically, is bad for us, but that gives us temporary respite or a way of expressing difficult emotions. According to this definition we all self-harm to an extent – drinking, smoking, drug-taking, eating foods of little to no nutritional value, starting a pointless argument with someone. They're all ways human beings have found to take the edge off the stresses of life.

"The thing that differentiates self-harm as a mental health issue is that it is usually done with the additional intention of self-punishment. So, we think of self-harm as something that happens when unbearable distress meets low self-esteem."

So, when you think about it, reaching for a bottle of wine and waking up with a banging head after a bad day at work is a form of self-harm, but it doesn't mean you have a mental health problem. We might be simply trying to numb the stress, forget about looming deadlines, perhaps even find some form of oblivion. But while this isn't particularly healthy, unless we're drinking to extremes or doing it so often that it risks job losses, it's not having a significantly detrimental impact on our lives. Let's face it, we're never going to be perfect little cherubs all of the time, shrugging things off with a sweet smile and an "oh well'".

But for some, self-harming behaviours become dangerous – even life-threatening – and this is often when they are part of a bigger psychological issue. It's therefore something we should always take seriously.

Nobody does it for a laugh.

you're so vain, I bet you think the chapter's about you

I've heard the words "egotist" and "attention-seeking" used about anxious people on more than one occasion. But there are two different drivers behind thinking that everyone should be talking about you.

The first is because you think you're worth talking about and people can't help but notice all your amazing attributes, talents and good looks. The second is because you think you're so [insert negative word here] that people can't help but notice how [insert negative word here] because you're possibly the most [insert negative word here] human being on the planet. You're basically preoccupied with how people perceive you – but not in a positive way – and you therefore seek reassurance.

Of course, there *is* the theory of narcissism (which is defined in the Cambridge dictionary as *having too much interest in and admiration for yourself*) – but things have to be pretty extreme to fall under that as an actual diagnosis!

Clearly, not all people seeking attention are raging narcissists (even though we can be pretty confident that all raging narcissists are seeking attention), but understanding the different types of narcissism reinforces the fact that it's difficult for us to make an assumption about somebody's personal drivers for attention unless we are a trained psychologist and they are our patient. We certainly can't make that assumption after simply reading somebody's tweets.

I first read about extroverted and introverted narcissism in *The Narcissist Test* by Harvard psychologist and *New York Times* bestselling author Dr Craig Malkin. I interviewed Dr Malkin to dig a bit deeper into these areas and to understand whether narcissism is, in fact, another area that is grossly misunderstood.

Dr Malkin said: "All narcissists are grandiose, not all are confident. Think of narcissism as the drive to feel special, exceptional or unique; there are many ways to feel special, and not all involve feeling like the richest or most attractive or brilliant person on the planet.

"We've identified three types of narcissism empirically: introverted (aka vulnerable or covert), extroverted (aka grandiose or overt); and communal.

"Extroverted narcissists are extremely confident. They're grandiose on the outside, thumping their chests and insisting they know better than everyone around them. Inside, however, they show signs of insecurity, specifically attachment insecurity – they don't trust that they can turn to people for comfort and care without being rejected."

In Dr Malkin's first example, it appears that narcissism serves as a kind of shield, a way of building a wall around a person's true vulnerabilities. It's as though they're sticking on a suit of inflexible armour to stop their tormented souls being exposed and prodded. I can see why it's incredibly difficult to empathize with a narcissist when all you're getting is what's being shown on the outside, but it's interesting to consider *why* somebody might behave in this way.

Conversely, as Dr Malkin went on to explain, introverted narcissists show the opposite pattern. He said: "They're insecure on the outside, self-doubting, hand-ringing and plaintive. They feel special by virtue of their suffering, agreeing with statements like 'I feel I'm temperamentally different from most people' and 'I have problems that nobody else seems to understand'. But inside, they're just as grandiose as any narcissist, hence the term, covert narcissist. They often secretly believe they're undiscovered geniuses. And whether they openly advertise it or not, they're certain they harbour more wisdom than the rest of humanity."

So, whether or not they are getting some form of attention from it, I'm not sure that either introverted or extroverted narcissism is a particularly happy place to be – for the person themselves and indeed for those around them ... And the third type?

Dr Malkin added: "Communal narcissists feel special by virtue of their altruism. They agree with statements like 'I will be well known for the good deeds I have done' and 'I am going to be the best parent on the planet'. They may or may not exude confidence, but they quietly adhere to the belief that their caring and support are beyond compare."

Communal narcissism reminds me of that episode of *Friends* – 'The One Where Phoebe Hates PBS'. Phoebe and Joey debate whether or not a selfless good deed can exist – because how is it selfless if doing something good (e.g. for charity) makes us feel good in ourselves, if we're getting some kind of emotional payback for it?

Of course, it doesn't mean we're all communal narcissists if we feel good about buying a copy of *The Big Issue* to support homeless vendors, or if we take part in a 5k run for a cancer charity. Like everything else, narcissism is on a spectrum and I can't see anyone being diagnosed as one just because they happen to have a lovely buzzy feeling wash over them when they make a charity donation. I mean, there's simply being human isn't there? We can enjoy that feeling and do good, but if we're desperate to be a world-renowned philanthropist for the odd good deed, if we're doing it *purely* for attention, maybe that's where narcissistic traits might really come into play.

restoring a sense of safety

Dr Malkin also agrees that not all attention-seeking is frivolous. He said: "The need for accolades and approval is wired into us and part of our developmental legacy. We can't develop a solid sense of self without some experience, as children, of feeling like even our crudest etching can earn a place on the refrigerator for all to see. By the same token, when we're in distress and fearful that our needs won't be met or, even more simply, when we need to know we're important to those closest to us, we're all prone to attention-seeking to restore a sense of safety."

So, needing attention isn't always about beating our chests and asking the world to fall to their knees in front of us. And, as Dr Malkin says, it's not even necessarily a choice but more a result of our evolutionary heritage – because we are social creatures who need connection to survive. In fact, without support, Dr Malkin says we can perish, stating research that has found loneliness to increase risk of death by a whopping 30 per cent.

the risks of having an attention-deficit

On the flip side, there is a risk involved in *not* seeking attention. Dr Malkin says this could be because of past experiences of being punished or criticized or abused for doing so. He said: "Those who don't seek attention also suffer. They tend to be more anxious and may suffer from depression. I call them echoists because, like their mythological name sake – the voiceless nymph who falls in love with Narcissus – they struggle to have a voice of their own and often fall into relationships with extremely narcissistic friends and partners."

So, some measure of attention-seeking is not only normal, but it is in fact *necessary* to our sense of safety and security in the world. Perhaps that is what is driving some of those posts we see, where an individual is tweeting about loneliness or depression. We might not ever know for certain, but maybe it's best not to judge?

But what harm is somebody causing to others if they are simply reaching out for attention – for support – because they're struggling? Why do they deserve our wrath? Our name-calling? Why should we try to shame them?

the impact

I asked people on social media about their experiences of being called an "attention-seeker" in relation to a mental health problem. Here's what they said:

"A senior A&E nurse called me an attention-seeker when I showed up as a teenager with a deep self-harm scar (on my thigh, where no one would see). I went home and cut myself again from the shame and anger of his words."

"I was called attention-seeking by friends, family members, teachers. I felt alone, beyond hurt, frightened and unable to talk honestly about how I was really feeling or ask for help. I still remember it and worry about it 15 years later. The way I fight that paranoia now is to speak openly about my experiences and normalize talking about mental health."

"From family members, there was 'stop pitying yourself' and 'get out of your head' and 'stop being so negative'. I felt shame and would partially believe the difficulty I encountered was my invention. I used to have negative self-talk that nothing good comes from speaking."

"During my stay in a psychiatric hospital, I overheard the nurses gossiping that I was only acting, seeking attention. I had to be put on heavy sedation and antidepressants (for the first time). I wasn't acting ANYTHING, except severely drugged. Part of me felt they were right, that I was a colossal waste of people's time and resources. The enduring part of me felt defiant. I'd overcome so much and needed help and how dare they be so damn unprofessional."

have I got your attention yet?

So what we know is that, for some people, needing the attention of others is part of their mental health problem. And rather than something to be judged, it is something to be understood and empathized with. But mental health problems and attention-seeking don't automatically go hand in hand. For some people, and I imagine more so with problems such as depression or addiction and some of the negative symptoms of schizophrenia, (i.e. social withdrawal), the last thing being sought is attention. And this is probably quite a dangerous thing, because mental health problems often thrive in isolation. The key is balance.

If you want or need some attention because you're struggling, or because you simply need a bit of validation for whatever reason, don't beat yourself up about it. It's normal – and it's necessary.

3

don't call me ... snowflake

I've always found it strange hearing people being labelled as snowflakes for standing up for their rights or for looking a mental health problem square in the eye. It makes about as much sense as a Matrix movie would to an audience of sleepy koalas after a heavy eucalyptus binge.

But where does the "snowflake" term even come from? As an insult, it's made its way into the *Oxford English Dictionary* where it is defined as: "A person mockingly characterized as overly sensitive, esp. one said to consider himself or herself entitled to special treatment or consideration."

In terms of modern-day use, an article in *The Conversation* from Shelly Haslam-Ormerod, a senior lecturer in mental health and wellbeing, states that the popularization of "snowflake" as an insult grew during the 2016 US elections as an attempt to shut down anti-Trump campaigners. And, sadly, it stuck – becoming adopted by anyone and everyone who felt unable to produce a coherent and reasoned argument in response to challenge (that's my view anyway). As well as those who, for whatever reason, simply can't face talking about mental health.

In the BBC's *Keywords For Our Time* series, writer Michael Rosen states that "snowflake" was used as early as the 1860s, where, in Missouri in the United States, it defined a person who was opposed to the abolition of slavery. An article in *The Week* explains the thinking behind this stating that"the implication of the name being that such people valued white people over black people".

It was also used in *Fight Club* – another brilliant but slightly confusing movie that would easily bamboozle a sleepy koala – and, if I'm honest, me. *Fight Club* was originally a novel by Chuck Palahniuk, in which he used the term "snowflake" as an insult more closely linked to today's derogatory usage. Palahniuk wrote:

"You are not a beautiful and unique snowflake. You are the same decaying organic matter as everyone, and we are all part of the same compost pile."

So, snowflake, as an insult, has some history, even though that history is inconsistent.

These days, however, the one consistent thing that runs alongside the snowflake insult is that it's always used to shut people down. It is usually directed at people who feel comfortable discussing matters of mental health or who demonstrate empathy. And it's usually delivered by those who, frankly, don't.

It seems to stem from a lack of understanding or willingness to engage in debate. It's like putting up a front to ward people off because, if they get too close and dig a little deeper, they might just realize that the person shouting "snowflake" has no argument at all. In fact, in my mind, calling somebody a snowflake comes across as being on a par with a toddler screaming "I hate you" because they've been caught stealing midget gems from the sweetie cupboard.

back in the day ...

We've seen the bullshit conversations about mental health where people have stated things like "Mental health didn't exist in the 1970s, we just got on with it" as though people didn't struggle because they were stronger "back in the day". All this stiff upper lip crap.

And it really is crap.

Firstly, given that everybody, without exception, has mental health, it's completely false to suggest that nobody had mental health in the 1970s/1960s/1800s/Stone Age.

Secondly, if they're talking about mental health *problems* not existing in the past, that's also entirely false and wrong. We might not have had the vocabulary to effectively articulate our mental health problems decades ago, and we were probably too afraid to talk about them because of the stigma surrounding them, but we definitely *had* them.

Hysteria, melancholy, opium habits weren't properly understood, but they definitely existed as a "thing" of their time. They were symptoms that probably stemmed from a mental health problem, or even a hormonal or physical condition that resulted in mental health problems such as depression or anxiety or addiction. Sadly, back in time, because understanding was so poor, mental health treatment and support was also poor – and we all know that there was a time when psychiatric hospitals were called asylums and people were generally locked up for having shed a few too many tears or for getting pregnant out of wedlock, or for some other ridiculous reason. Nobody wanted to be "committed to an asylum". So, I'd argue that it's unlikely people "just got on with it" in previous decades. I'd suggest they struggled enormously, were incorrectly diagnosed and/or self-medicated.

In my view, people didn't used to be "stronger" when it came to their mental health in previous decades – they just tended to keep quiet about it. I certainly did in the 1990s when I first began to experience panic attacks. People didn't talk about mental health as much then, so the only people I spoke to about these weird, crushing, terrifying episodes were my mum, my doctor and my therapist. My friends didn't know – even though, as I've since discovered, a few of them were experiencing panic attacks at the time as well. We were all far too ashamed to tell each other.

Oh, and we didn't have Twitter then either. So, no 1970s or 1980s or 1990s children would broadcast about their mental health, what they ate for tea, who killed Bobby Ewing, whether or not they cried over Scott and Charlene's wedding or to wish a #Happy30thBirthdayMadonna. All our conversations happened behind closed doors – or in print. And, unless you were an elusive *Dallas* character or

Kylie and Jason, you were hardly likely to make the pages of *Hello!*.

Being more proactive in managing your health is, undoubtedly, a strength – and that includes talking about it openly too and being a leader in the conversation. It's funny that, although we are accepting of how other things have changed since the 70s or 80s, such as our over-reliance on Findus Crispy Pancakes and bright blue artificial food colouring, we don't belittle people for now choosing to eat fresh and opting for more natural foods, do we? We understand that, through science, we've learnt that there are better choices we can make to prolong our lives. So why can't we see mental health in the same way? If we are proactively making choices about our mental health that can help us to live stronger, happier, longer and more resilient lives, how on earth does that make us "weak" or "snowflakey"?

Why is taking control considered meek and feeble? It's entirely nonsensical. And the only logical explanation I can come up with is projection ... perhaps those who are criticizing this proactive approach to mental health are projecting their own fears onto others.

making the headlines

When I think of the "snowflake" label, the use that immediately springs to mind comes from the UK tabloid newspaper, the *Daily Star*, which, in 2018, ran with the following headline:

SNOWFLAKE KIDS GET LESSON
IN CHILLING

It was about a school that was running mindfulness classes for pupils. So, if we explore the paper's logic, what they're saying is that kids who take self-defence classes for the mind to stave off mental health problems, kids who learn disciplined and proven new skills to add to their armoury, they're saying those kids are … weak?

Would you say that about Rocky Balboa's training sessions? Is he less of a hero because he trains before a match?

I'd take a punt and argue that no, he certainly is not. In fact, if he didn't train before a match, and headed straight into the ring unprepared, he'd be kind of stupid and probably not come out of it all that well. We'd no longer be singing "Eye of the Tiger", we'd be lamenting the fallen hero with a Celine Dion ballad. *Rocky* would be some obscure film from the 1980s that nobody really bothered with at the time, let alone talked about in 2022.

And while we're on the subject of recent times, it hasn't exactly been a walk in the park has it? We're living in a world where right-wing politics has gone completely off the scale, Brexit is causing all kinds of chaos, we're in the midst of a climate change emergency, racism is both inherent and broad-daylight-brazen in society and we're emerging slowly, anxiously and uncertainly from a pandemic. Add to all this the fact that many mental health support services have been cut and we've got the perfect recipe for adversity and distress.

So surely, if teachers are helping kids develop the skills they need to keep their brains match-fit and deal with all this shit, that's a good thing?

Author and mental health campaigner, Natasha Devon MBE, through her Mental Health Media Charter initiative, and with a boatload of support from many mental health and education influencers, slammed the *Daily Star* for its use of the headline and the damage that it could have on those it was ridiculing, reminding us all that the article was about *primary school children*. And after numerous letters, including one directly addressed to the editor, and a tonne of tweets, the *Daily Star* refused to reply.

Who're the snowflakes now?

"Flakenstein"

British tabloid *The Sun* churned out the snowflake insult on its front page in 2018, apparently irked by the idea that English Literature students today sympathize with Frankenstein's monster and instead see him as a "creature" and a "victim".

Firstly, duh! As comedy writer Aaron Gillies (aka TechnicallyRon) tweeted in response to this story: "Snowflake students claim Romeo and Juliet may have had 'problematic' relationship'."

It's hardly groundbreaking – even if the trend is, as the English Literature professor, Nick Groom, stated, shifting more toward sentimentality for the "creature".

Secondly, how and why does understanding literature deem you a snowflake? Again, this comes back to bored people (and newspaper editors trying to appeal to them) trying to get a reaction for attention (or sales) and feeling out of touch with current views or conversations.

And if we're leaning on the "empathy" part of the story, well, my God, how does it make you weak or over-sensitive to have enough depth that you can find empathy for others?

I mean, in baby boomer times gone by, when Mick Jagger had sympathy for the devil, nobody called him a snowflake did they? No, instead, he was accused of being "evil", the devil himself and a part of the occult (as Jagger discussed in a *Rolling Stone* magazine interview).

Funny how times change.

"Feeble"

In a piece for the *Daily Mail*, Claire Fox, head of a think tank called The Institute of Ideas (which sounds to me like a spoof source from *The Daily Mash*), discusses "Generation Snowflake". When writing about her experience with A-Level students in 2016, she described them as a "fragile, thin-skinned younger generation".

Fox stated that, when she was in the school, debating the controversy around footballer Ched Evans, who was at the time convicted of rape (and later cleared of the charge) she provoked anger, challenge and tears when she stated (in her own words as reported in the *Daily Mail*):

"I dared suggest (as eminent feminists have before me) that rape wasn't necessarily the worst thing a woman could experience."

Firstly, there is no "worst thing", and, secondly, what if one of these young women *had* been raped or sexually assaulted? What if they *knew* someone who had?

So, these young women, for feeling empathy, for speaking out and challenging this viewpoint, are considered snowflakes? Really?

"Wrapped in cotton-wool"

In late 2019, UK tabloid the *Express* ran a piece focused on Piers Morgan's calling out of the "snowflake generation", and his assertions that kids today have never had it so good and are being wrapped in cotton wool. The article also included Morgan's comments on how "anxiety-ridden snowflakes" are too quick to dwell on the negatives of life.

Hang on a minute: these so-called "snowflakes" are the ones facing up to the fact that mental health problems are very real and, in some cases, fatal. They are seeing them, talking about them and dealing with them. I would argue that, if they were wrapped in cotton wool, they'd simply be sticking their fingers in their ears and refusing to talk or act upon this stuff.

Kids have never had it better? Well, how do we define better? Is convenience *really* better? The Kristof column that Piers is quoting from talks of running water and electricity. Sure, that's great. I'm glad I don't have to wash in mucky puddles, warm myself by a bonfire and empty a piss pot out the window into the street below. But life isn't black and white. Convenience, as we can clearly see, takes other valuable features from our lives.

If we're hard-wired to hunt for food, or sit around campfires with our neighbours sharing stories, then removing all of that from us is bound to have an impact on our wellbeing. We simply don't communicate in the same way that we used to thanks to digital technology. When it comes to anxiety, we often hear the term "fight or flight" because, regardless of whether or not we're being chased by a tiger, we have that inbuilt response mechanism and it sometimes goes into overdrive. This means that, although our everyday stresses are not, for example, fearing we will be eaten by a literal tiger, as they were for our ancestors, our in-built response mechanism doesn't know that they are no longer a threat, and so it can sometimes go off in the same way, making us feel overwhelmed. Of course, because the threat isn't literally there, we don't have to "run" like our ancestors did and we are therefore unable to get rid of that adrenaline. It stays with us. But also, just because the tiger isn't *literally* chasing us, it doesn't mean there isn't a metaphorical tiger that's just as threatening and potentially damaging on our tails.

If anyone's wrapped in cotton wool, I'd say it's those people who bury their head in the sand with regards to mental health problems. The ones who pretend it doesn't exist or that it didn't happen in the 1960s/1970s, etc. Because it did! We've just got the language to articulate it better now, and more clinical and medical expertise to help us through it. The contributing factors aren't "all better" than they were – they're just different.

the impact

I spoke to people on social media about their experiences too. Here's what some of them said:

"When I was involved with a pro-wrestling organization, I requested to take some time away to look after my physical and mental health and was subsequently ridiculed in front of the entire locker room, told to 'man up' and called a 'snowflake'. The wrestlers would make comments on social media too about their former 'snowflake ring announcer'".

"I get called a snowflake by my brother all the time because I'm a feminist who advocates for things. He is massively against that so he uses that word to make me feel weak and powerless."

"I get called a snowflake often by my nan if I dare mention I'm going through a low patch (ironically she is now heavily depressed and expects understanding). Her usual reasoning was that I had nothing to be down about."

"I've been referred to as a snowflake for suggesting that someone in a comments section should consider the mental health of the person they were piling on. Apparently it's silly and unnecessary to consider the effect of online abuse. It just made me angry that it seemed so unreasonable to remember that people on the internet are real people behind the screens."

resilience

In my opinion, the "snowflakes" being labelled as such aren't "weak" or "over-sensitive". Cast your mind back to the 1970s punk movement. The activism, the taking no bullshit, the calling out of bad politics, the protesting ... how is that different to today's young people standing up for themselves and for others? Young people who are keen to make change happen and to create strength and resilience through learning, developing and not sweeping things under the carpet and hoping they'll go away?

On the topic of mental health resilience, someone once said to me on Twitter: "If a child falls off their bike, tell them to get back on." Well, yes – that's not a bad idea. But if they get back on with a helmet and an increased awareness of road safety, they'll stay on that bike for longer, surely?

Resilience comes from learning, not ignoring. It's just a shame that so many people misinterpret what resilience *really* means and where it comes from. It certainly doesn't come from closing your eyes, clicking your heels together and repeating "There's nothing to be scared of" three times over. It comes from facing what's out there. It comes from facing whatever challenges are in front of you by acknowledging them. Chasing an unhealthy resilience stereotype, which might involve ignoring problems and therefore not attempting to deal with them head on, is going to see you eventually fall to your knees.

Author and mental health campaigner, Natasha Devon MBE, said: "People tend to talk about resilience as though it's a character trait, or an attitude an individual can choose to switch on or off. It's become this aspirational thing – 'Ooh look how resilient I am' – and it's tied up with some of the more toxic offshoots of capitalism, like praising people who overwork, or thinking its virtuous to be stressed."

I think we've all seen examples of that – like who can stay latest in the office to feel validated, worthy and show themselves to be "kick-ass hardcore"? Who can keep going the longest?

The problem is, you might keep going the longest in the short-term scenarios you're currently focused on, but are you *really* going to be able to keep it up in the longer term? There's got to be some serious wear and tear involved in that kind of approach. So how does it possibly make you stronger?

It's like jumping in the pool and going like the clappers for the first few lengths before dragging your sorry arse out the water early because you think you're about to have a heart attack …

Ultimately, you lose.

What does resilience actually mean?

There are many different ways to describe resilience – it's not exactly black and white. But one thing it clearly isn't is burying your head in the sand and pretending everything's OK when it isn't.

If your engine management light comes on and you think it's no big deal, that it's probably just an issue with the electrics, and therefore you ignore it, you could well end up back in the car sales room forking out another fortune. Because it wasn't a superficial problem with the dashboard – your cooling system was fucked and, while it was crying out for some care and attention, you kept going, causing your brand-new motor to overheat, conk out and end up in the knacker's yard. And your bank balance is now in the red ...

Anything you think about in life – be it a car, a house, a human being – if it doesn't get serviced and supported, one day it could well become unserviceable.

Natasha said: "In my experience, resilience is actually a by-product of being well supported. The more meaningful connections you have in your life, the more resilient you'll be."

This takes us back to the previous chapter on attention-seeking, and the fact we're hard-wired to have (and to need) social interactions. A result of having those social interactions, communication outlets and wider support is resilience.

We can also look at how self-care and healthy boundaries support our resilience. As mental health nurse and campaigner, Cara Lisette, said: "We learn ways to manage adverse events and feelings from early childhood and there are various things over our lifetimes that will lead to us developing variable levels of resilience that are likely to fluctuate. We learn resilience from our parents, our friends, the media, health professionals. I know my resilience to cope with stress and difficult situations is hugely reduced if my mental health isn't where I'd like it to be and if I am burned out. Knowing this, as I have got older, I am learning much more about how to say no and how to look after myself."

What might cause a resilience deficit?

There are a few combinations of behaviours that reduce our resilience capacity. As Harvard psychologist Dr Malkin puts it (quoting renowned psychologist, Fosha) "feeling without dealing" is the first. He said: "Feeling without dealing tips us into disruptive emotion displays that erode rather than foster closeness."

I think what Dr Malkin is getting at here is that if we try to shut things off, if we don't address them and simply choose to ignore them, they can erupt into angry or distressing outbursts that cause more problems.

He added: "Meanwhile, dealing without feeling makes us seem cold and unapproachable, also eroding the support and care we need to stay happy and healthy.

"Finally, feeling and relating without dealing leaves us hopelessly dependent on others, with little sense of confidence or agency."

So, it really is a holistic mix of our own willingness to acknowledge and deal with the challenges life throws at us, self-care tools, social support systems and an ability to tap into our emotions.

And while it might be considered "brave" or "strong" to simply tap into the things we can do *alone*, lack of social support can radically reduce our levels of resilience.

Dr Malkin added: "Those of us raised with the trust that when we're sad, scared, blue or lonely we can turn to one special person or a special group of people who will be there for us, no matter what, for mutual care and comfort, develop attachment security – and regardless of genetics, it's clear that feeling secure in this way blesses us with resilience: securely attached people comfortably explore the world, seek out and maintain closeness, and can express and manage emotions."

The tree metaphor

Positive psychology practitioner and trauma-informed coach, Ruth Cooper-Dickson uses a brilliant metaphor for resilience. She said: "In terms of the *types* of resilience there are three – and I like to use the tree metaphor.

"Firstly, we have a palm tree. It blows about wildly in the storm but when the storm passes it bounces back to its original position. This is called bounce-back ability.

"Secondly, we have the old English oak, which represents stoicism. Life can throw lots at us but we don't move or get shifted in the storm. When the storm passes, we are the same as we always were.

"But then we have a third metaphor. Imagine any kind of tree in a storm getting struck by lightning. This is like being really badly knocked by an adverse life situation. The tree gets broken and splintered. After a time, flowers begin to sprout and we see new shoots of growth. This is basically a metaphor for post-traumatic growth. This doesn't happen every time we are shaken badly, but this shows how trauma can change us."

Ruth explained that the idea of these three types of resilience is that we are not always the same type of tree throughout our lives. She added: "While our childhood experiences and personality style do affect our propensity to deal with challenges – and there is certainly a nature/ nurture thing to consider – there are actually factors based on what is happening at the time that affects resilience levels. For example, is there support available? Are you living somewhere safe? Do you have a strong sense of purpose? Are you in a position to use your self-care toolbox? Our ability to be resilient does come down to this constellation of factors."

I asked Ruth a bit more about this, particularly enjoying the tree metaphor. I wanted to know, if the tree was protected from the elements by a strong wall or a fence, what might happen if that wall or fence one day fell down, and the tree was then subject to a storm.

Ruth said: "I think there are two things that could happen here. Firstly, we might find that the tree has been so well protected that it can't navigate any difficulty at all – a small storm will really knock it, never mind a hurricane. This is about being over-protected or too wrapped up. But it might also be because some people simply do not experience as much difficulty in their lives as others – whether that be because they have a strong family unit, a good start in life, no traumas or adversity, etc. And the result might be the same – a storm could really knock them.

"If we weather the storm, we develop coping mechanisms – and they might be either good or bad coping mechanisms. But either way, we can learn from them. We can understand what works and what doesn't. And that makes us more resilient.

"The second option might be that the tree has been well-protected but, if we think of the wall as the parents, what happens if those parents do protect their child but at the same time, teach them about the storms, and teach them about the tools they may need to cope. So, when that wall comes down, they are well prepared. They are resilient."

I found this fascinating because it goes back to that Daily Star headline about the "snowflake kids" getting "lessons in chilling". The teachers were acting as their "wall" (and we must remember we are talking about very young primary school children) but teaching them the tools they may need for the day that wall crumbles down. For when they become independent.

This way they will become stronger – and more resilient.

a dangerous term

Undoubtedly there's a big problem with the term snowflake – the assumption that people talking about or focusing on their mental health are weak and, as we've seen, it is most often used by a bunch of angry people projecting their own shortcomings onto others.

But why does it matter?

One former mental health nurse who contacted me said: "I think nowadays it diminishes people's beliefs, makes them feel as if their beliefs are not valid or they are trying too hard. It can affect people's feelings of self-worth, self-esteem, make them question their views/place in the world."

Being called weak or over-sensitive if you are struggling with a mental health problem could make you think twice about speaking out or asking for help. And that is when it becomes dangerous.

If you believe that people are going to ridicule your concerns, why would you put yourself through it? Even though today, we are more aware of the different kinds of mental health problems and have the language to describe what is happening to us, it still isn't *easy*. You start questioning yourself – maybe I *do* need to just pull myself together? Maybe I *am* being over-sensitive? Maybe I'm just a weak person?

Before you know it, because you haven't been able to embark on the road to recovery, your problems get worse. Not only that, your self-esteem and confidence plummet because you believe all these awful things about yourself – that you're weak and over-sensitive. That adds *even more* pressure to your mental health. Soon, your low self-esteem and mental health problems are in cahoots, hitting the mosh pit of a death metal gig and violently shaking even more health and happiness out of your tree.

You keep going to school/college/work because, well, you're not *really* ill are you? You're just a weak person. You're just being over-sensitive to your emotions. So, you go in. And having to sit in meetings or exams when you're not on top form, and having to put on a front and make excuses for why your concentration is all to pot or you're tired all the time, is absolutely draining. Exhaustion and stress are now chucked on top of that mosh pit and the shaking continues, with the big booming death metal soundtrack thwacking your brain until you're plunged into …

See where I'm going? If you don't feel able to stop and say, "I'm not OK right now, I need some help", then you're eventually going to hit the floor. But the truth is, recognizing that you're not OK and asking for help, these are real strengths. They show that you're not afraid, that you're refusing to bury your feelings and that you aren't afraid to look directly into the eyes of your problems. It means you're kick ass, basically. It means you've got your game face on.

After all, no respected sportsperson looks away from the ball. The only way to win at wellbeing is by keeping an eye on your mental health.

In summary, snowflakes are beautiful phenomena. Collectively, they create a powerful avalanche. On the other hand, red-faced, angry people just create spit.

4

---

don't call me ...
miserable

We often use the word "depressed" to communicate feelings of fleeting sadness. Perhaps your team's conceded a point, or you missed out on tickets for Glastonbury or Coachella? Gutted!

But it's more a disappointment than anything else.

Conflating feeling a bit down with diagnosable depression is problematic – not least because it belittles the challenging experiences that so many people go through. As with anxiety (more on that later) it confuses everyday responses and feelings with a mental health problem – and the difference is stark.

While we might all feel sad from time to time (and sometimes that sadness can be crippling), if it's relative to the situation and it passes swiftly, then it is unlikely to become an enduring and diagnosable mental health problem. That doesn't make acute sadness an easy ride of course – within those parameters we might have grief or separation – not just a low feeling about the break-up of some pop band. Such experiences can be incredibly challenging and, in some cases, may well persist and develop into a mental health problem such as depression.

According to Mental Health America, symptoms of depression include:

- Persistent sad, anxious or "empty" mood
- Sleeping too much or too little; middle of the night or early morning waking
- Weight fluctuations; reduced appetite and weight loss, or increased appetite and weight gain
- Loss of pleasure and interest in activities once enjoyed, including sex
- Restlessness, irritability
- Persistent physical symptoms that do not respond to treatment (such as chronic pain or digestive disorders)
- Difficulty concentrating, remembering or making decisions
- Fatigue or loss of energy
- Feeling guilty, hopeless or worthless
- Thoughts of suicide or death

As you can see, not all of these symptoms equate to sadness and yet sadness (or feeling "blue", "miserable", "down in the dumps", whatever you want to call it) is often described as feeling depressed.

Conversely, because of this association, when somebody is *actually* depressed, they might all too often be confronted with words like *"cheer up, it might never happen"* or *"snap out of it"* or *"put your game face on and stop being so miserable"*.

However, if you are suffering from depression, there's more going on in your brain and your body than sadness and therefore a more complex approach to treatment and recovery is often required.

Mental health nurse and campaigner, Cara Lisette, told me that depression can develop from sad events but also for no rational reason whatsoever. She said: "Factors that lead to people experiencing depression are multifaceted. It is absolutely possible to experience depression as a reactive response to challenging life situations, such as poverty, grief and relationship difficulties. However these factors can be dynamic and not everybody who experiences difficulties in their lives will become depressed. It is equally the case that depression can be diagnosed in people with no obvious external influences. Mental illnesses are complex and everybody's experience will be personal to them."

Cara's explanation gives us greater insight into why the question *"but what have you got to be depressed about?"* isn't helpful. And while we might feel frustrated that someone seems "miserable" and we can't see any reason behind it, we need to remember that depression is a reason *in its own right*.

On the other hand, people with depression might not appear sad at all. In fact, you might see smiling selfies on Instagram and they might laugh at your bad jokes. This doesn't mean they are "faking it" when they tell you they are depressed. Behind the scenes, they could be experiencing a crushing emptiness, a debilitating sadness or a range of other symptoms such as fatigue, lack of motivation, inability to concentrate, sleeping too much or too little and so on. And if we go to the extreme end of the spectrum, there also may be no clear outward signs that someone is feeling suicidal. This is why checking in on someone and listening without judgement is paramount. Sometimes people are very good at masking what's going on inside.

So what's the impact going to be if we tell somebody with depression to "stop being so miserable, take a walk and get over it"? Cara's heard many of her patients describe how it makes them feel. She said: "Telling someone with depression to 'cheer up' is completing invalidating. There are absolutely things that people can do to help themselves, and there are interventions for depression that can be very successful. Depression does not have to be a lifelong illness and many people can recover with the right support, but the right support is key. There is no illness in existence in which 'snapping out of it' is an effective treatment."

the impact

I asked people who have experienced depression or significant life trauma how it has made them feel or act when somebody has told them to stop being so miserable. Here's what they said:

"I was told 'you better stop looking so fucking sad as it's making me look like a bad supervisor' by someone whose bullying caused me to leave my PhD. It made me feel like every part of me was under their control and belonged to them – even my facial expressions. Less than two weeks after that exchange I attempted suicide."

"I've been asked, 'You've got depression? Doesn't mean you have to be miserable about it though. It's not just an excuse to stay in bed is it?'"

"Someone told me they didn't understand why I didn't just get over it. They said they had had a bad day a few months before and they went for a long walk and watched an old film then felt a lot better. I had no words. I had severe depression and I wasn't able to attend university, wash, eat or leave my bedroom. It was extremely frightening and it felt like such an insult when she said that."

"'Smile more', 'Cheer up', 'It can't be that bad' and the ones who try to be 'funny'. 'Ohh someone's looking miserable!', 'Who died?', 'Aren't you Mr Cheerful today?'. Thank you, random stranger, my suicidal thoughts are all gone because of your hilarious words. I'm cured, what a miracle."

"I was told, 'You don't look depressed, you always smile when we see you in meetings'."

happy pills

One stereotype commonly associated with depression (and anxiety in many cases) links to the medication used to treat it. At the time of writing this chapter, I've been on antidepressants for almost eight years. And I should make something very clear … I'm not enjoying a relentless rave in my living room with saucer eyes and glowsticks. In fact, I've just been quietly watching a YouTube documentary on how the ancient Egyptians built pyramids … This idea that drugs for mental health problems – particularly depression or anxiety – are "happy pills" is really not based on anything.

But antidepressants certainly aren't innocent little candy pills – they change what's going on in your brain after all, so they're a serious business. But when you are struggling significantly with mental illness, they can really help you to get back on track. And this is why stigma and scaremongering is problematic. The tabloid newspapers shouldn't be telling us what medication we should or shouldn't be taking – this should be part of an open discussion with a health professional where questions can be asked, answered and considered. But if we are bombarded with stigma, reaching that informed discussion point might not happen because our minds might already be made up …

Antidepressants are interesting because they have different effects on different people and it's pretty impossible to 100 per cent prove what they are doing to your brain. Some people feel well and stable on them, whereas others might experience anxiety or suicidal thoughts. But for individuals who are really struggling, with the right support from your doctor and your loved ones, antidepressants could save your life.

There are lots of myths and complexities surrounding psychiatric drugs – from antidepressants to anxiolytics, and from mood stabilizers to anti-psychotics. For this chapter, however, I'm going to focus on antidepressants simply because the stigma surrounding antidepressants (particularly the "happy pills" idea) seems to reach huge numbers of people through tabloid headlines (even hitting the front pages).

it isn't right or wrong to take antidepressants

I'm neither a relentless cheer leader for antidepressants nor somebody who believes they are the root of all evil. For me, they work – but for others, they can be detrimental. I can share my own experiences up until this point, but I haven't yet tried to seriously taper off them. I therefore have no idea if stopping will be a walk in the park or a bumpy ride on the road to hell. All I will say is that, aside from a rather unattractive increase in sweating (yuk), they've worked pretty well for me so far. My moods are pretty stable (at least, compared to what they were before) and my relationships with family and friends are more balanced too. I started taking them to put a stop to the panic attacks (antidepressants can be prescribed for both depression and anxiety), but the positive effect

I experienced was broader – somehow, I feel as though antidepressants have given me the time and space to think before I react (badly) to life.

how do antidepressants work?

I asked psychologist Dr Helen Casey to explain how the most common form of antidepressants in use today – SSRIs (Selective Serotonin Reuptake Inhibitors) – work. Dr Casey said: "SSRIs are a class of antidepressants developed in the 1970s and '80s. It's not known exactly how they are effective but the predominant theory is that they work by increasing levels of serotonin in the brain. Serotonin is known as one of the body's naturally occurring feel-good chemicals associated with enhanced mood, better emotion regulation and improved sleep. So higher levels of serotonin in the brain are thought to ameliorate some of the symptoms we see in depression."

So, they increase serotonin which is thought to make us feel better. But how do they do it? Dr Casey said: "Serotonin is a neurotransmitter that carries signals between nerve cells in the central nervous system including in the brain. During signalling, serotonin is released and then reabsorbed and recycled – a process known as re-uptake. SSRIs act by blocking re-uptake, which increases the amount of serotonin available for transmission of signals to neighbouring nerve cells."

When serotonin levels are too high or too low, mental health problems can occur. Both serotonin and another neurotransmitter, noradrenaline, are linked to mood and emotion. But the key thing here is that people do not take antidepressants to have a *high* mood, they take them to *normalize* their mood, which is very different to getting off your face on illicit drugs on a weekend. It's about levelling, not flying.

when are antidepressants prescribed?

Dr Casey explained: "SSRIs are prescribed as a first-line treatment for major depression and a second-line treatment for less severe depression that has persisted for some time and is resistant to other treatments, such as talking therapies. On average it takes up to four weeks to become fully effective. As well as depression it is used for a wide range of other conditions including anxiety, PTSD, OCD, phobias, panic disorders, eating disorders and some pain disorders. There is also evidence that SSRIs can help improve mood swings in Borderline Personality Disorder. It is also related to a difficulty in ejaculating both during sex and masturbation, and for this reason it is sometimes prescribed for premature ejaculation."

If anything can suggest that antidepressants aren't "happy pills", I think Dr Casey's last statement about premature ejaculation does! If they're stopping you from reaching orgasm too quickly, then surely they're playing down the ecstasy somewhat, not driving it up! Indeed, as Dr Casey explains, the side-effects include reduced sex drive, so …

do antidepressants really work?

The reason there is a lot of seemingly non-committal language around how antidepressants work (i.e. they're *thought to* …) is because it's not actually possible to measure your neurotransmitter levels like you can measure other kinds of hormones.

For example, I have a thyroid disorder and have to have yearly blood tests to measure the levels of the thyroid hormone in my blood. My medication is adjusted according to the results and my symptoms. Some people with a thyroid deficiency may have low levels but no negative symptoms, and therefore their doctor may decide they don't need medication. But some people can have borderline low levels of thyroid hormone *and* experience symptoms of a thyroid disorder. In this case, like me, you might be given meds.

With antidepressants, doctors are only able to go by your symptoms. There is no test to measure how much serotonin you started with, or how much serotonin you now have since taking medication. It's all about impact – are the meds helping to relieve your symptoms? If so, they're doing their thing and working well for you.

Dr Casey said: "Evidence for efficacy is mixed. For example, some studies have shown no statistically significant effect for those taking SSRIs compared to placebo in mild to moderate cases of depression. However some evidence suggests SSRIs appear to be particularly effective for those with persistent depression when combined with CBT or other psychotherapies, possibly because patients are better able to access talking therapies when their symptoms of depression are less prevalent."

So, when it comes to antidepressants we can see that they work for some people. And how they help can vary too – some might benefit from taking antidepressants for a brief period as they enter talking therapy. Others, however, might take them longer term as I have. It's very much a personal experience but, as Dr Casey mentions above, seeing medication as *part* of the bigger picture for mental health treatment is going to be more effective than using them in isolation.

the risks and side-effects

As with any medication we might take, SSRIs do have side-effects – some severe some less so. Dr Casey explained: "SSRI side-effects might include, for example, nausea, agitation, insomnia, emotional blunting, reduced sex drive or erectile dysfunction. They are also sometimes associated with increased self-harm and suicidality among those under 18 years of age and for this reason SSRIs are rarely prescribed for this group. There is some evidence to suggest an association between SSRI use and aggression but there is a lack of consensus in the literature.

"Coming off SSRIs is also associated with adverse withdrawal symptoms – for example anxiety, nausea, flu-like symptoms, seizures or dizziness, and for this reason stopping is safest when it involves reducing the dose in stages under the guidance of a medical professional."

As one of those patients who likes to read the pill packet leaflets from start to finish, I also know that it is widely understood that taking too much of an SSRI can lead to serotonin syndrome, which is a potentially serious side-effect that causes confusion, sweating, shivering, diarrhoea and many other symptoms. What it *doesn't* do however is get you energetically dancing on the spot to Josh Wink's "Higher State of Consciousness" for 12 hours flooded with so much ecstasy you'd consider Brexit a good idea.

antidepressants are not magic bullets

It's worth highlighting that antidepressants rarely work in isolation – doctors usually prescribe them as part of a more holistic approach to managing a mental health problem. So, you should never be given a pill and told to be on your way – there should be regular contact with your doctor to review how they are affecting you, as well as discussions around talking therapy, diet, exercise, social support and more. Plus, as already mentioned, they're not always used to treat depression alone – they can be prescribed for a range of anxiety disorders too, including Generalized Anxiety Disorder, PTSD and OCD.

Family doctor Dr de Giorgio explains how and why she might prescribe somebody antidepressants: "I would say to patients that antidepressants are just one of the tools we have to help them manage their depression/anxiety or both. We would use them when a patient is too unwell to manage their usual life in the way they need/want to or when they are a risk to themselves. Ideally all patients would have early access to high-quality talking therapy first, but waiting lists are often months and, sometimes, where a patient is too poorly, there could be a risk of harm if they wait. So, I may start the medication to keep them safe, but work on getting those talking therapies as well, as this is how people get better faster and, importantly, stay well longer term too – by learning coping mechanisms and better understanding their experiences of trauma, for example."

Dr de Giorgio admits that doctors would probably provide fewer antidepressants if there was better access to different types of talking therapies of a decent duration. She added: "The obsession with six sessions of CBT to fix everything means that not everybody gets the therapy that they need."

the impact

I asked people about their experiences of taking antidepressants and how stigma or a lack of understanding had impacted their decision-making. Interestingly, I didn't receive a single response that said, "they made me high" or "they made me elated." The "happy pill" idea certainly doesn't ring true when you hear real experiences. But the responses were incredibly varied. Below are a selection of experiences that people shared with me.

"I have taken an anti-depressant for about seven years. I was apprehensive about starting it, partly because of the perceived

stigma of being unable to cope without drugs and partly for concerns about side-effects. They have been extremely effective for me – I would describe the effect as preventing my mind from spiralling downward into catastrophizing and self-hating thoughts and making me much more able to deal with day-to-day life. I am not keen on being dependent on anti-depressants for the rest of my life, but each time I have tried to come off them, however gradually, I have found my troubling thought-patterns and suicidal thoughts recur, so for the moment I am continuing on my low dose."

"My early perception of antidepressants was they don't work, and I was initially really hesitant to go on them as I thought they'd somehow make me weak for needing to take them. Six years on and, although I've had to change the type or dosage over the years, they allow me to function daily and they keep the worst thoughts away."

"People always implied they would make me feel 'fake happy' but that is crap – they make me feel less awful and more stable. They're not happy pills – I'd call them 'not crying every morning before 7am for no apparent reason' pills."

"I wasn't enthusiastic about taking them due to the stereotype. None of them made me 'happy', they just took the edge off the awfulness. They left me 'flat', no real ups or downs. They allowed me to continue to function, but I'd be lying if I said I was 'living'."

"I felt like a failure for needing them and for not being able to 'pull myself together'. They seemed like a crutch I shouldn't need. I was brought up on the 'life's a bitch and then you die' mantra, *suck it up and get drunk to relieve the pain. I felt like taking them was admitting that I was mad, that there was something wrong with me, something that was my fault, that I should've been able to do something about."*

"The stigma I encountered from my ex about taking antidepressants was bad. He told me that if I took the medication it meant that I was in no fit state to be a parent. Luckily my doctor was amazing and helped me realize that it was in fact the opposite – I was showing strength and commitment to being a good parent by taking action."

This chapter isn't designed to suggest that anyone should or shouldn't take antidepressants. This is a highly personal decision that should be made in conjunction with a health professional. It is also not suggesting that antidepressants will or won't work for people – we are all unique and therefore likely to respond differently. For some people, they are lifesaving; for others, they are detrimental.

What this chapter is arguing against, however, is the idea that antidepressants are some kind of "happy pill" – some kind of low-level high wrapped in prescription medicine packaging. This couldn't be further from the truth.

5

don't call me ... workshy

From: r.snotty@anyjob.com
To: i.judge@anyjob.com
Did you hear? Zoe from admin's meant to be off sick, but Sarah from accounts said she spotted her in Starbucks.

From: i.judge@anyjob.com
To: r.snotty@anyjob.com
No way! I fricking knew it! Dan from IT told me it was meant to be depression. But if she's in Starbucks having a mocha, she's blatantly skiving.

From: r.snotty@anyjob.com
To: i.judge@anyjob.com
Never mind the mocha. She was spotted with a chocolate muffin too. And, OMG, you'll never guess what else ... she was only with her sister! Brazen cow. Anyway, fancy a long lunch tomorrow? The boss is out all day ...

Office gossip. If we haven't heard it, we've definitely *imagined* hearing it when we've needed time off for a mental health problem, and the things we might need to do to recover might be the very things we're scared of doing for fear of being "found out".

If you have a mental health problem such as depression, for example, has anyone ever told you that drinking a latte, eating cake and chatting to friends and family will set you back? Hell, no! In fact, you're more likely to be prescribed those things than told to avoid them. However, while the majority of employers these days promote their support of mental health campaigns and provide counselling services or Mental Health First Aid training, stigma around time off for mental ill health still persists. And where there isn't a genuine culture of support and understanding, employees pick up on this and either get caught up in presenteeism (showing up to work, regardless, when they're unwell, or simply feeling the need to stay late and be seen as a hard worker – therefore contributing to a potential mental health problem or at the very least stress and exhaustion) or feel unable to speak the truth about why they need time off.

Dr Stephanie de Giorgio, a GP, told me that because the variety of physical and mental illnesses is so huge, and because there is such a crossover between them, it's difficult to say you might be prescribed "x" for a mental health issue and "y" for a physical health issue. However, she also said that it's probably more difficult for somebody with a mental health problem to rest, eat and sleep because the people around them might not be as accepting of them doing so, compared to if they were struggling with a physical illness.

In fact, Dr de Giorgio has had personal experience of this. She said: "Patients do get nervous about doing the right thing for themselves – and even I have struggled myself. The only time I was off work with mental illness, I remember being so worried about being seen meeting friends for coffee or taking a walk by the sea, in case colleagues saw me and thought I was skiving. I have often had discussions with people about holidays when signed off with mental illness. It may be exactly what they need, but many are worried it will be taken badly. And I can't lie, some people may see it that way. The same goes for physical illness sometimes, but a lot less than for mental illness."

Dr de Giorgio says she hopes that this is improving, because, ultimately, being able to do the right thing for your own wellbeing is paramount. But this is precisely why we need to talk about this – to challenge the "skiver" perception of those who need to take time out from the pressures of work to recover. Frankly, I can't imagine that there's any better respite than reading a book on a beach …

So, what is the impact of stigma on absences relating to mental illness?

presenteeism

One problem that needs to be addressed to ensure that people with mental health problems aren't discriminated against in the workplace is presenteeism. Ruth Cooper-Dickson, a positive psychology practitioner, has spent years working with big corporates and smaller organizations to review workplace culture and embed more positive approaches to wellbeing. She told me: "Presenteeism is an issue that we find in many workplaces. I was personally working in a culture of presenteeism when I worked in Asia. There was a 'first in, last to leave' kind of culture, and you'd certainly not be expected to leave the office until after your boss did. That was eleven years ago and, thankfully, things have changed. But they're certainly not perfect."

I'm sure many of us have experienced this at some point. I worked for one organization where several of us regularly stayed behind after hours purely to prove to the boss that we were wholly committed to our jobs. It made us feel that we were part of the hardcore grafter gang of office troops who were tough and resilient and would keep going relentlessly because nothing was as important as the day job.

Of course, this is another example of the misconceptions surrounding resilience. Your resilience won't thrive if you keep ignoring what your body and brain needs and, ultimately, you'll become less productive in your work. Unfortunately, however, too many of us, even if we don't like to admit it, still believe that working all the hours available to us is evidence of resilience and being good at our job.

If you were sitting in the office long after the sun went down, chatting to the boss about non-urgent stuff (when you *really* wanted to be at home eating pasta and bingeing on *Succession*), you felt that you were more likely to go somewhere. Especially since your more sensible colleagues who clocked off at 5.30pm were often discussed in a disparaging fashion after they had left the office …

But, on reflection, I see this kind of managerial brown-nosing as slightly embarrassing and a total waste of time. There's nothing hardcore about brown-nosing. It reeks of desperation. However, sadly, in some workplaces, it's still the thing to do to secure your position and future prospects. But how can this be good for your health – or for the business?

According to the Mental Health Foundation, 1 in every 6.8 people (or 14.7 per cent) in the UK experience mental health problems in the workplace. The Foundation also states that 12.7 per cent of all sickness absences in the UK can be attributed to mental health conditions. But you have to wonder how accurate this figure is, because, due to the pervasive "snowflake" stereotype relating to mental health, how many people are actually citing mental health when taking time off for that reason? And, to be clear, I'm not just talking diagnosable mental health conditions here. Stress must also be acknowledged as, if left unchecked, it could lead to a diagnosable mental health problem too. In fact, in a 2022 report published on Mental Health America, entitled *Mind the Workplace*, 4 in 5 employees reported that workplace stress affects their relationships with friends, family and coworkers – clearly evidencing how stress impacts their lives outside of work.

Even as somebody who was openly blogging about living with an anxiety disorder, there were times when I would report the physical symptoms of my mental health problem rather than the condition itself. I've called in sick with stomach problems before, which I did have, but they weren't caused by a dodgy takeaway or gastric flu; they were caused by my anxiety. I just never mentioned that bit. It seems ridiculous that I was far more embarrassed about having a problem in my head than I was about having the shits. How does that make any sense?

Mental health campaigner and founder of youth mental health charity, Beyond, Jonny Benjamin MBE, told me that he has also downplayed his mental health problems in the workplace. He said: "Presenteeism was a particular issue when I worked in television a few years ago. The job was extremely high pressured and resulted in a lot of anxiety and stress. One day I had a panic attack at my desk while on the phone to a particularly rude client. Afterwards, I would have regular panic attacks in and around the office. It was a horrible experience and I'm not sure how I sustained it for so long."

This is one of the key recurring issues that goes hand in hand with panic and anxiety. Sometimes it's the fear of a panic attack, as opposed to what has driven the panic in the first place, that is the most problematic trigger and you can become stuck in a loop.

I personally experienced this when I worked in theatre. I've always had an irrational fear of peeing myself in public and that became a big part of my anxiety. Once, at an all-staff meeting, a rush of panic suddenly flooded me and, convinced I was going to flood the theatre foyer, I legged it to the loos.

Once I'd associated this type of panic with this particular scenario (i.e. a big meeting), I struggled to contribute effectively in future all-staff meetings because of my preoccupation with needing the loo. Even smaller details could trigger this fear, such as the kind of seat I was sitting on at the time (since that meeting almost 20 years ago, I've avoided z-shaped bar stools at all costs).

Jonny's panic attacks resulted in regular sickness absences, but, like me, and no doubt many others, he always cited physical health issues as the cause, instead of being honest about his mental health difficulties.

Looking back, I think that if I had been able to openly say what was triggering my panic attacks, I'd have been less likely to experience them. It's the shame and the sheer effort it takes to literally sit on the attacks, in the hope of snuffing them out, that causes the panic to build in the first place.

Thinking back to chapter 2 on attention-seeking, it sometimes feels as though we are attention-seeking if we talk about how we feel *psychologically* in a moment. It's not as seemingly tangible as a physical health issue, such as needing to leave the office because you feel sick, so we keep shtum. But this only results in more attention being drawn when the panic decides it's time to break loose, bursting out of you like the Incredible Hulk. We've denied ourselves a release valve so Vesuvius blows and our adrenaline and cortisol is visibly spewing out all over the place. And then, guess what? We feel even worse and even more worried about it happening again.

But we can't create these release valves in isolation. They are only effective if the workplace genuinely embraces mental health support.

you can't change culture with a hashtag

Let me start by saying I have seen some great examples of supportive workplace cultures and I've also experienced some great ones first hand. But many toxic and stigmatizing workplaces still exist. And, of course, there are also those in the middle – employers that want to do the right thing, but are still on a bit of a steep learning curve.

A few years ago, I was invited to give a talk at the CIPD's (Chartered Institute for Personnel Development) AGM about mental health in the workplace. I've spoken in many workplaces about mental health stigma, but for this event I decided to focus on culture specifically.

One of my slides was entitled "You can't change culture with a hashtag" because I'd seen this happen far too often. Organizations shout about supporting #WorldMentalHealthDay or #TimeToTalkDay, they might sign the Time to Change Employer Pledge with a nice photo op, and they might provide counselling. But counselling services aren't adding value if a poor workplace culture is what's driving the need in the first place …

What I mean by this is that, while a workplace can *say* it embraces mental health support and that it tackles stigma, if the core culture is toxic and/or if the leadership team isn't genuinely behind it, then it simply can't happen. Additionally, the mental health services provided by the company might be mopping up the impact of a bad workplace culture, rather than adding value – they might simply be serving as damage limitation tools.

Jonny Benjamin has given many talks in companies and been approached afterwards by many people who said they felt unable to be honest with their employer about their mental health problems. He said: "Currently, I see mental health as a tick box exercise for too many organizations. They will mark events in the calendar such as World Mental Health Day or organize a few of their staff to do Mental Health First Aid Training, but that is often as far as their commitment will go. Nevertheless, I do feel that the pandemic, in spite of all of its damage, has forced some workplaces to really focus on the mental health of staff."

So yes, it is good – brilliant in fact – to have support services and campaigns on the go. But if employees feel unable to share their mental health struggles, or if they feel discriminated against, then the problem is in the fabric of the organization – and that's not a quick fix.

If employers are genuinely keen to transform workplace culture and effectively support colleagues' mental health, then it is something that can – and should – be addressed. It just needs investment and some brave and bold conversations to take place from the top down.

stand up and be ... shamed?

On more than one occasion, I experienced toxic culture and discrimination when I was employed as part of an in-house team.

One example was being marked down in an appraisal for "unprofessionalism" for challenging workplace culture in a staff survey team review session. The session was introduced as a safe space to be *totally honest* about what it was like to work for the company. I suggested that we needed to look at culture, not just support services. I was later told that this was deemed unprofessional as I was a line manager ...

Another example was when I had a phased return to work after extended sick leave. I'd had what my doctor described as an "acute stress reaction" and anxiety. My return-to-work interview, which was supposed to be supportive, was a bit of an unwelcome surprise to say the least. A member of the HR team was there (I wasn't warned about this and it wasn't common practice) and the words "performance review" were used. I'd never had any issues prior to being off work with mental health issues in any of my appraisals.

This company was especially vocal in its support of mental health and of tackling stigma, and yet my first day back in the office after one of the most challenging periods of my life was met with an informal performance review, and an accusation that I had been off doing other things and leaving my colleagues to "pick up the slack".

The company was talking the talk but not walking the walk.

the impact

I asked people on social media to share their experiences of workplace discrimination or lack of support relating to mental health problems. I've included a small handful of responses below:

"My doctor suggested I ask for a day a week working from home to cut out some of the stress while I was struggling with my mental health. Management said no and suggested I go part time. After this my boss started treating me differently – asking for examples of my work, suggesting that others were covering for me. There had been no issues with the quality of my work prior to my mental health disclosure. I'd lost my job because I was honest about my mental health."

"I had a major mental breakdown due to a family crisis that put me under a lot of pressure. I was off work for six months and when I returned I was immediately put on a capability plan (also known as a performance review). It was presented to me in a meeting that had been described as a 'wellbeing' meeting, but it just turned into a discussion about my capability."

"I told my new line manager about my depression and soon after things started to go downhill for me and I found myself being criticized regularly. The right things were said – she would ask 'How can we support you?' but no support ever materialized. Struggling with depression, alongside a couple of significant physical health problems, I was afraid of being seen as incapable so forced myself into work every day when I was actually incredibly unwell. Eventually, both my physical

and mental health declined significantly. At that stage I was referred to occupational health, who seemed to suggest that perhaps my physical problems were blown out of proportion by my depression. It felt to me that, in saying I had depression, I was saying that my judgement couldn't be trusted. I kept forcing myself into the office until, one day, feeling desperate and anxious, I stood at the top of the stairs and wished I had the strength to throw myself down them, just so I didn't have to go in. I realized how serious things were, saw my doctor and was immediately signed off."

---

employers and managers need support too

If the leadership of an organization is toxic and averse to authentic mental health support, things can be difficult for both employees and line managers – and HR teams too. But there are also times, particularly within smaller organizations, when the employer wants to do the right thing but feels lost and unsure about how best to help.

I heard from one former line manager who said he felt really concerned about a relatively new colleague who was struggling at work. The manager discovered that it was the anniversary of the employee's mother's death – she had taken her own life and the employee was understandably traumatized by having found her. The manager was worried about how best to support his employee, particularly after he shared his feelings of suicidal ideation.

The manager said: "I didn't know what to do so I wrote to his GP, explaining the situation and how concerned I was. They informed me that they couldn't do anything – moreover, they couldn't discuss a patient with me due to confidentiality. I totally understand that – it's fair enough. However, if they could have even just signposted me to some information or guidance that would have been really helpful. But I was given absolutely nothing."

shifting cultural norms

Ruth Cooper-Dickson told me that she has seen some strong examples of organizational culture genuinely embracing workplace wellbeing, rather than just paying lip service. She said: "I went to Asia recently and a manager told me that they always made a point of standing up in the office at 5.30 pm, announcing they were going home and encouraging their colleagues to clock off as soon as they could as well. It's like a stance against presenteeism – and it gives colleagues permission, as well as a more senior role model, which is important."

So, in addition to "role-modelling" and setting good examples, what else can managers do to encourage a healthy workplace culture? Ruth said: "Having managers who are competent and able to having coaching conversations with their employees is important. It's not just about having performance reviews, but about being able to understand and coach a colleague effectively, so they can be their best self. Relationships need to be built on trust, and we also need to stop de-prioritizing one-to-ones and check-ins – we should make a commitment to never, where possible, bump them out of the diary. Encouraging and giving permission for colleagues to attend wellbeing events is also key – and this should also be role-modelled by the line manager as well. At the end of the day, burnout will decrease productivity, and a healthy workplace will increase it, so it's definitely worth investing in."

It might sound as though I'm diving into productivity, services and support rather than stigma at this point, but investing in wellbeing events and prioritizing one-to-ones are all about ensuring that employers marry what they say with what they actually do. If these activities and services aren't truly embraced, then there is probably some inherent stigma lurking within the organization and the culture of the company. And this isn't necessarily about lack of technical mental health knowledge, it's about understanding and empathy. Big shifts need to take place to encourage safer and more productive environments that truly support people with mental health problems.

how to support colleagues with mental health problems

After leaving television, Jonny Benjamin went on to work for the national mental health charity, Rethink Mental Illness. He said: "On my very first day in the office my line manager sat down with me and together we filled out a WRAP plan, with sections included within it such as such as 'What signs can we look out for if you're struggling?' and 'What can we put in place for you if you're feeling unwell?'"

WRAP – or Wellness Recovery Action Plan – was first developed in 1997 in the US, a collaboration between several dozen individuals who had experienced serious mental illness, including facilitator Mary Ellen Copeland, now a renowned author, educator and mental health recovery advocate. The plan, which is today a part of the Advocates for Human Potential, Inc portfolio, has five key principles: hope, personal responsibility, education, self-advocacy and support. It helps people to support their goals and achieve and maintain wellness.

Unfortunately, not long after beginning his new role with Rethink, Jonny suffered a relapse in his mental health. However, this supportive workplace culture meant he was able to continue going to the office. He said: "My incredible line manager, Peer, who I am eternally grateful for, saw the signs that I was becoming unwell and put the WRAP into place. This meant that I was now doing things a little differently, such as avoiding the rush hour when coming into or leaving work, and taking my lunch break away from my desk while doing something like taking a walk outside. All staff at Rethink Mental Illness filled in a WRAP and the result was a much more open, honest and supportive workforce than I'd ever experienced before."

I think that a WRAP, due to its formal nature, provides a way in which we can stop stigma (to some extent anyway) in its tracks. If these agreements are written up and put in place, then there is evidence that the employer has agreed to take mental health seriously and that, in doing so, they agree to do x, y and z. It makes things more practical and more likely to be taken seriously.

Going back to the stats on the Mental Health Foundation website, it states that better mental health support in the workplace can save UK businesses up to £8 billion per year. And Jonny's experience is a good example of why this is – because with a few minor adjustments, he was able to continue being a productive and effective team member.

A flexible return to work

Another misconception about mental illness and being "fit for work" is that it's an all-or-nothing state. You might be able to quietly get on with desk work, for example, but find meetings difficult. Or, as Jonny described, you might find travelling to the office during rush hour problematic.

I know from times that I have been off work with severe anxiety that participating in creative meetings or presenting to senior colleagues was something I felt unable to do. When I first returned to the office, my brain wasn't working quickly enough and I felt that I was too distracted to string a coherent sentence together.

I think what this also shows is that it isn't about simply being present in the office – about whether or not you can physically make it into the office. It's about the *types* of activities that your brain can process effectively, without being detrimental to your recovery.

Mental health days

One of the new "perks" we see being promoted by employers is mental health days. On the surface, these sound great, but in reality could they be causing more of an issue? I spoke to Bernie Wong, Senior Manager of Insights and Principal for US-based workplace mental health non-profit, Mind Share Partners. Bernie has previously written about the pros and cons of mental health days for Forbes, and I think his views on the topic are well worth consideration.

Bernie told me: "At the individual level, mental health days offer protected time to relieve built-up stress and anxiety from work, as well as time to reflect, reorient and take care of personal matters outside of work. My biggest issue with mental health days is when they are positioned as a wellbeing strategy, absolving companies of their own responsibility in creating healthy and sustainable cultures of work. Sky-high work demands, poor work-life balance, unsupportive management, emails late into the night – there are countless work-related factors that can cause mental health decline, proven by research. Mental health days don't solve any of these things, and over-reliance on mental health days, without addressing our culture of work, simply creates toxic cycles of burnout."

Some of the research Bernie is referring to dates back several years, long before mental health days were even a "thing", so this link between work stressors and mental health decline has long been known, even if we're only *just* starting to address it more proactively. However, looking at one of the more recent research papers he shared with me from JAMA Psychiatry, we can see that for individuals with an existing diagnosed mental health problem, psychosocial stressors at work can increase the risk of decline and related absence (the risk was up a whopping 76 per cent among workers exposed to these stressors compared to those who were not).

Other research Bernie points to, such as a paper in the Scandinavian *Journal of Work, Environment and Health*, demonstrates how work stressors can not only worsen *existing* mental health problems, they can also *cause* some of the more common mental health disorders.

From this we can see that, although mental health days may give an individual a short period of breathing space, they aren't addressing the *cause*, therefore leaving at-risk individuals in a perpetual revolving door of sickness absence. A sticking plaster, in some ways. So, while this doesn't *on the surface* appear to be about stigma, in many ways it is. An over-reliance on benefits like mental health days shows a lack of understanding (or lack of willing in some cases) to properly address workplace wellbeing and acknowledge mental health problems as a serious risk to employees. You could argue, in the case of individuals who are struggling, that it's the equivalent of someone with depression being told to "go for a walk" to get over it. Yes, that might help to a degree, but *never* in isolation.

Of course, this is not to suggest that mental health days are a bad thing, but they need to be used *appropriately*, as part of a more holistic approach to workplace wellbeing. Bernie added: "Mental health days should be used proactively; to create flexibility for individuals to navigate the unavoidable or the unforeseen – not as a release valve for fundamentally broken or exploitative cultures of work.

Leverage mental health days proactively and intentionally. Plan them after seasonal crunch times or company-wide to send an organizational message. Offer flexibility in when and how they're used. And establish norms around work leading up to, during, and coming back from time off."

I think the key message here is that mental health days should be considered a "perk" and nothing more. They *do* add value, but they should be part of a broader approach to support and they should *never* replace time off for mental ill health, which should always be treated on a par with time off for physical ill health.

those caring for people with mental health problems

While we often focus on the person experiencing the mental health problem directly, we need to remember that caring for somebody with a mental health problem can also be traumatic and stressful. And it can, in fact, create poor mental health in the carer. Jonny said: "Something that is often forgotten about in all this discourse is the mental health of the carer. I have spoken to many carers of parents, spouses, children and other loved ones whose wellbeing is often impacted but overlooked within their workplace, and indeed the rest of society.

"I'll never forget talking to a senior member of staff within a law firm about being the sole carer for his wife who was struggling with depression at the time. He felt that he couldn't be open about his situation at home with any of his colleagues at work, despite it having an increasingly detrimental effect on him."

So, this highlights another area in which we need more understanding. But given that we still have a long way to go in terms of genuinely empathizing with colleagues who are off with a mental health issue, it strikes me that it could be some time before carers of people with mental health conditions are taken seriously. Perhaps this is where some of the more forward-thinking, progressive organizations can take some bold steps and share some best practice.

where can we go from here?

While some companies are doing really well in this area, there still appears to be an issue with employees feeling that they can confidently and safely tell their employers when they are off work with a mental health problem. There is a fear of not being believed and concerns about feeling ashamed. And as Dr de Giorgio, a GP, has said, this kind of corporate stigma and self-stigma will actually inhibit our recovery.

The most difficult part of the problem is workplace culture. No matter what benefits or policies an employer has in place, the core beliefs held by senior leadership will ripple throughout the organization and impact all colleagues. But as employees we *can* start to chip away at this ...

I've known colleagues take suggestions to HR or management about introducing a wellbeing group. This can create a safe space for a group of colleagues committed to mental health and wellbeing to work together to make positive changes. It means that no one person need put their head above the parapet because you're working as a team.

Additionally, as Jonny mentioned, a WRAP plan can help to document and formalize agreements about the support you might need, making sure that these things *do* happen and that line managers feel more confident in knowing how to help.

Any individuals concerned about workplace culture, mental health discrimination or a lack of support might also find it helpful to get to know who their union reps are and explore whether a membership might be helpful. Then, should you ever feel that you are being discriminated against, you have a representative to support and advise you.

But probably most important of all, make sure that, as colleagues, you're there for each other. There's nothing worse than feeling alone when you're struggling with a mental health problem. Even in organizations that aren't providing adequate mental health support, just having a peer to confide in, and knowing you're not alone, can make a huge difference.

So, let your colleagues know you're there for them. Let them know that you understand and that you don't judge. And if someone takes time off for mental ill health, do exactly the same as you would if it were a physical health issue. A card, a text or a bunch of flowers will remind them that you care.

6

don't call me ... psycho

What's the first thing you think of when you hear the word "psycho"? Norman Bates, perhaps? Blood-curdling cries and spatter in a shower cubicle? *Killing Eve's* Villanelle choosing a stylish new costume and calmly travelling the world to kill people in a myriad of novel ways?

There's a boatload of connotations surrounding the word "psycho" which, as a prefix, precedes many well-known, but not so well understood, conditions, states or treatments including (to name but a few):

- Psychosis/psychotic
- Psychopathy/psychopath
- Psychotherapy
- Psychoactive
- Psychology

And then, just slightly out of sync (without the "o"), we also have psychiatry …

"Psycho", however, is often used as an insult to describe someone experiencing any manner of debilitating or severe mental health problems. It's as though the more you struggle, the greater your vulnerability, the more flack you're going to get.

Conversely, it gets used flippantly too (think "he's acting a bit psycho" when a friend is a bit wound up or edgy), again reinforcing the stigma.

The definition of "psycho" in the *Oxford English Dictionary* is: "Relating to the mind or psychology." However, you don't have to look too far down the Google list of dictionary definitions before you come across all manner of descriptors:

- "A crazy or mentally unstable person."
- "Someone who has serious mental problems and who may act in a violent way without feeling sorry for what they have done."
- "A psycho is a deranged or psychopathic person."
- "A psycho is defined as someone or something that is crazy or insane. Stalking your ex-lover and killing his family pet is an example of behaviours that would be described as psycho."

You can see why this is problematic. Because out of the words I mentioned above that begin with the letters P S Y C H O (and believe me, there are *many* more), most have no correlation to violence and therefore should not instil fear at all – yet they often get jumbled up and confused.

Of course, you might be a *little* apprehensive about your first *psychotherapy* session, for example, but you wouldn't expect your psychotherapist to stalk you or murder your pet. And neither should you expect somebody with *psychosis* to stalk you or murder your pet but, sadly, this fear persists. And research shows that psychosis is one of the most stigmatized of mental health problems.

On the other hand, *psychopathy* genuinely *can* be associated with violence and fear. This isn't to say that somebody with psychosis absolutely will not cause harm to another or indeed that somebody labelled as psychopathic absolutely will, but what we need to understand is that, just like some people who drink can become abusive, the majority do not. And we can say the same about psychosis. As somebody once said to me, people experiencing psychosis are more likely to be afraid of the world than the world should be of them.

When British spy thriller *Killing Eve* (which I loved, by the way) was first screened on BBC America/BBC Three in 2018, I saw tons of social media posts and articles talking about the cool and ruthless assassin Villanelle, as being "psychotic". But Villanelle is far from psychotic. She is quite likely *psychopathic*. The two are completely different.

So, this chapter will focus on the significant difference between the two diagnoses, explore the character of Villanelle as a case study, and discuss why it's dangerous to get the two words muddled up.

what is psychopathy?

Using the character of Villanelle, we can begin to understand what the classic traits of psychopathy are. If you haven't come across this lead character in *Killing Eve*, let me explain. Played by actress Jodie Comer, Villanelle is a cool, calculating and charming assassin – with a penchant for quirky and luxury fashion. She plays by her own rules, enjoys acting out different characters as part of her meticulously planned-out killing missions, and has a cheeky and endearing side that viewers adore. *But* she is a cold-blooded killer – and her empathy levels are firmly in the red. Well, bankrupt might be more accurate as I don't think we really see her display any, even toward Eve, who she develops a bit of an obsession with. So, is Villanelle a psychopath?

Dr Luna Muñoz Centifanti, a psychologist and Honorary Research Fellow at the Sir Arthur Institute of Social and Economic Studies (University of West Indies in Jamaica), knows a thing or two about psychopathy and she told me how the character of Villanelle relates to the diagnosis. She said: "The character of Villanelle displays classic psychopathy traits. There is a debate on how many factors there are in psychopathy, but some of the classic ones are: callousness, manipulation, antisocial behaviour and lifestyle choices, and criminality.

Dr Muñoz Centifanti explained that we can see all these traits in Villanelle, regardless of who she's interacting with. So, whether it's the victim of one of her killing missions, the professional relationship with her boss or the potential of a romantic relationship with Eve, she is still showing callousness and manipulation and lying to get what she wants. But are all psychopaths violent?

Well, it depends on how you look at it. Dr Muñoz Centifanti believes that while some people may display psychopathic traits they might not necessarily be physically violent with people. But their behaviour in corporate or governmental roles could have the potential to indirectly cause violence in other ways.

She added: "If you classify violence in terms of physical violence and murder directly, OK not all psychopaths will engage in violence and murder. But people with strong psychopathic traits may be emotionally violent, for example, causing pain in others in different ways."

so, what is psychosis?

I'll start by saying it couldn't be further removed from psychopathy. Unfortunately, due to the connotations around the term "psycho" and the huge misunderstanding around psychosis, which is less an illness in its own right and more a problem associated with many states or diagnoses, many people who have experienced psychosis have felt ashamed or isolated and afraid to seek help.

According to UK mental health charity, Mind, psychosis is "When you perceive or interpret reality in a very different way from people around you. You might 'lose touch' with reality ... The most common types of psychotic experiences are hallucinations, delusions and disorganized thinking and speech ... Psychosis affects people in different ways. You might experience it once, have short episodes throughout your life or live with it most of the time."

Breaking it down further still, let's look at what these different psychotic experiences might entail.

- **Hallucinations:** This might involve seeing or hearing things that others can't or experiencing tastes, smells or other strange sensations with no apparent cause. Hearing voices, for example, could be positive and helpful or hostile and nasty.
- **Delusions:** This is when you believe in something that has no real foundation – for example, there might be delusions of grandeur (e.g. believing that you're rich and powerful or that you can read minds) or paranoid delusions (believing that everyone is out to get you).
- **Disorganized thinking:** This might include racing thoughts and ideas, speaking very quickly, finding links that don't really exist and struggling to concentrate.

Can you imagine being able to carry out a ruthless assassination like our anti-hero Villanelle, while experiencing psychosis? Planning the logistics of the perfect murder, disguising your guilt, covering your tracks and keeping your designer clothes blood spatter-free, while your brain is simultaneously flitting from one thing to another and racing at a thousand miles an hour? I can't see this being possible let alone likely. I'm not suggesting that experiencing psychosis could *never* lead to violence, or that violent people are somehow immune to psychosis, but one thing is for sure, Villanelle is not psychotic – and psychosis *does not* equal violent.

Millions of people around the world get wasted on a Saturday night, but we're not afraid of them all. Even though there are gazillions of people whose minds aren't especially clear or rational, there is only a teeny percentage who cause havoc or behave violently.

Why might this be? In some cases, possibly because they're total arseholes even when sober, and the booze is just releasing a concentrated, uninhibited version of what already exists. Of course, in some individuals, out-of-character behaviours can happen under the influence. But why should we be more scared of one person in a room who happens to be experiencing psychosis, than a hundred people in the pub who've drank a bottle of Prosecco each? It doesn't make any sense. I've been threatened by drunken people, I've been hit by drunken people, but I've never been threatened or attacked by anyone experiencing psychosis.

Maybe it's because I've been drunk many times myself. It's familiar to me. Maybe the fear of psychosis comes from the unknown? Perhaps we are just scared because we don't understand psychosis and what it *really* is? Perhaps we confuse psychosis with personality defects? But psychosis is an experience that so many people completely recover from. And I don't believe that the onset of psychosis has anything at all to do with personality traits ...

schizophrenia

Even though there are many different causes of psychosis, schizophrenia is often one of the first things we think of when we talk about psychosis.

Before we go on to discuss the wider causes of psychosis, we'll explore schizophrenia in a little more depth because, just as psychosis is hugely misunderstood, so too is schizophrenia, which many people mistakenly believe is like having a "split personality" (it isn't).

In 2019, I was involved in some research on behalf of St Andrew's Healthcare, a charity that operates many psychiatric hospitals and services around the UK. They wanted to understand stigma in relation to serious mental health problems, such as borderline personality disorder and schizophrenia. I was working for NewcastleGateshead Initiative at the time, a public-private partnership organization that, in addition to its place-based work also had a commercial research arm. My colleagues and I designed and carried out the research on behalf of St Andrew's and the results were significant. A whopping 58 per cent of respondents believed that schizophrenia meant having a split personality. Additionally, 12 per cent believed it's "when somebody is a psychopath" (again reinforcing the need to make a clear distinction between psychosis and psychopathy).

The study also found that, while 50 per cent of respondents would try to talk to someone they knew if they were diagnosed with depression, only 24 per cent said they would do the same if they knew someone diagnosed with schizophrenia. And 27 per cent would be nervous of someone with schizophrenia, compared to only 5 per cent with regards to depression.

But it's interesting to note that, while many feel frightened of people with schizophrenia, they don't actually know what it is.

So, what really *is* schizophrenia?

According to the charity Mental Health America, schizophrenia is "a serious disorder that affects how a person thinks, feels and acts." The charity goes on to say, "Someone with schizophrenia may have difficulty distinguishing between what is real and what is imaginary; may be unresponsive or withdrawn; and may have difficulty expressing normal emotions in social situations." Mental Health America lists the following symptoms:

Positive symptoms (disturbances that are "gained"):

- **Delusions**: false ideas – for example, individuals may believe they are being spied on.
- **Hallucinations**: seeing, feeling, tasting, hearing or smelling something that doesn't really exist.
- **Disordered thinking and speech**: moving from one topic to another in a nonsensical fashion.
- **Disorganized behaviour**: having problems with routine behaviours such as hygiene or choosing appropriate clothing for the weather.

Negative symptoms (capabilities that are "lost"):

- Social withdrawal
- Extreme apathy
- Lack of drive or being inactive
- Emotional flatness

I also know from the research I was involved with that many people feel scared to talk to people living with schizophrenia, but this creates problems as the person experiencing it is likely, at times, to be vulnerable and in need of support.

According to the World Health Organization (WHO), schizophrenia is an illness that affects around 20 million people worldwide, and people with schizophrenia are two to three times more likely to die early than the general population. The WHO also states that "People with schizophrenia are prone to human rights violations both inside mental health institutions and in communities." It states that this in turn can "limit access to healthcare, education, housing and employment."

So, there's very clear evidence of vulnerability and, while addressing stigma alone won't solve the many problems faced, it might at least influence societal support and understanding in the community, which would surely make a big difference. There are often arguments put forward that we need to move away from anti-stigma campaigns and focus all our efforts on funding and service provision, but I believe the two are inter-linked. For example, stigma can influence a community's response to a proposed psychiatric facility, directly affecting service provision.

I've seen this happen when local residents, no doubt unsure of what schizophrenia and psychosis really mean, have petitioned against supported accommodation being built in the locality for people with severe and enduring mental health problems (many of whom had schizophrenia). I spoke to the individuals using the service after their new accommodation was successfully built, and the effect this community outcry had on them was palpable. The shame they felt for being considered "a danger to society" was a significant blow to their self-esteem and wellbeing.

what else causes psychosis?

While schizophrenia is possibly the most well-known cause of psychosis, even though it's probably one of the most misunderstood of mental health problems, there are many other causes.

Dr Jess Heron is a senior research fellow in perinatal psychiatry with the University of Birmingham's Institute of Mental Health, and CEO of the charity Action on Postpartum Psychosis, a UK organization that exists to support women and families affected by postpartum psychosis (PP). This debilitating illness affects around 1,400 women each year in the UK and around 140,000 women around the world.

Postpartum psychosis is a frightening and debilitating illness for mothers and families. It is important to note how it differs from postnatal depression, as many mothers with PP do not experience any symptoms of depression, rather they experience extreme elation, spirituality and confusion, and lose contact with reality.

Dr Heron told me that psychosis can occur as part of a number of mental health problems including bipolar disorder, severe depression, schizophrenia, schizoaffective disorder, borderline personality disorder, addiction and withdrawal – and even illnesses like obsessive compulsive disorder can be experienced to a delusional intensity. She said: "The postpartum onset of psychosis seems to be most closely linked to bipolar disorder. Women with bipolar disorder are at particularly high risk of experiencing PP, but many women who experience PP haven't had any previous mental illness. They may, however, remain at risk of illness at times of great hormonal change – after birth, and during menopause."

Dr Heron explained that, according to research, childbirth is the most potent known trigger of psychosis, and there is a 22-fold increase in the risk of psychosis in the days or weeks following childbirth compared to any other time in a woman's life. This relative risk increases to 31 times when comparing first births only to any other time in a woman's life. As PP can occur in women who have had no previous mental health problems, it is important to understand the role biology plays in psychosis.

Dr Heron said: "The causes of postpartum psychosis are not well understood, but the fact that it runs in families suggest that genes may be important, and the close relationship between symptoms and the large biological and hormonal changes that occur at birth suggest for some people that their vulnerability to psychosis may be linked to their reproductive hormones. Social and psychological factors appear less important in the onset of PP compared to other forms of psychosis. Social class, education level, financial circumstances, the baby not being wanted or lack of partner support do not seem to be involved in causing PP. The jury's out on birth trauma and mode of delivery, but first delivery, sleep disturbance and pre-eclampsia may play a role."

Dr Heron speaks to hundreds of women who have experienced postpartum psychosis and says there is still a significant stigma surrounding psychosis that causes distress and pain for many women and families. In fact, according to The Confidential Enquiries into Maternal and Child Health (MBRACE-UK), suicide is the leading cause of maternal death in the 12 months after childbirth. Dr Heron added: "Up until the launch of the APP charity, half of these suicides were to women experiencing postpartum psychosis. We have done a great deal of work to raise awareness, and increase the amount of support and information available to women and families in the UK. The proportion of maternal deaths due to PP is now much reduced, but PP must always be managed as a medical emergency. The risk of harm to mother and infant are very real because of the rapidity and severity of symptoms. Lack of awareness, shame and stigma still stop women from seeking help when they most need it." Due to this stigma, many women and families fear contact with mental health services, because of concerns about their child being taken away from them if they ask for help. This delays treatment and puts mum and baby more at risk. But Dr Heron told me that, in reality, the UK has excellent facilities for supporting new mothers experiencing psychosis, with specialist facilities and expertise, enabling mums and babies to remain together during treatment. These specialist services are called Mother and Baby Units and they provide excellent care for many families, however, sadly, there still aren't enough of them around the UK.

This is why APP supports women and families to tell their real-life stories of postpartum psychosis in the media to tackle stigma, campaign for more specialist services and broaden understanding. Dr Heron added: "Public understanding is key to good outcomes, enabling women to get help quickly and face less trauma during recovery. Misinformed and sensationalist media stories cause fear for women and families. Women with PP need urgent care to keep themselves and their babies safe. In the extremely rare occasion in the UK that a mother slips through the net, it is a failure of our systems and our society that will have an impact for generations to come. The MBRACE-UK statistics evidence this."

So, it's fair to say that psychosis isn't fussy about who it affects. It does not discriminate, can sometimes have hormonal or biological causes and, in many cases (especially in the case of postpartum psychosis, which is eminently treatable) people can and do make a full recovery.

media portrayals of psychosis

Action on Postpartum Psychosis has worked closely with TV producers, filmmakers, authors and theatre practitioners to bring authentic stories to life in creative ways. This is an area of work that the UK charity Mind has also been involved with for many years through their media advisory service, which was initially set up by former journalist Jenni Regan.

Thankfully, and no doubt because of the dedicated work charities are doing in this area, media representations of psychosis are becoming more and more responsible, and the awareness-raising media work that often takes place around such storylines helps audiences to understand the issues in even more depth.

However, going back to the research I mentioned earlier carried out on behalf of St Andrew's Healthcare (see page 105), there is still a need for more mental health portrayals, especially with regards to the more stigmatized of mental health problems such as psychosis. As part of that survey, we asked respondents to name a fictional TV or movie character who has experienced a mental illness. As part of the response to this question, Norman Bates of the movie *Psycho* was identified as having schizophrenia. He does not.

Other harmful portrayals have been seen in the music industry. Kasabian's "In Love With a Psycho", and accompanying video released in 2017, showing a bunch of people dressed up and pretending to be psychiatric patients was heavily criticized by many in the mental health community. At the time, I wrote a full comment piece for *Standard Issue* magazine on the topic, and Sue Baker OBE spoke out on behalf of Time to Change, the UK's national mental health stigma-busting movement. Sue argued that, although there was probably no intent to cause harm or insult, and that there may have even been a degree of irony in what Kasabian were attempting to do, the end result was nonetheless harmful. It reinforced age-old tropes about psychiatric hospitals and pushed the "psycho" stereotype into the mainstream. According to Wikipedia, as of late 2021, the music video has been viewed over 13.8 million times on YouTube, so this just shows how powerful creative media and the arts can be in either challenging or reinforcing harmful stereotypes.

"Sweet But Psycho", released in 2018 by US artist Ava Max, was another controversial song with an accompanying music video and stigmatizing imagery. Again, there was the argument that it had a deeper meaning, that it was about gaslighting, but the use of a padded cell, and the association of violence and mental illness, all combines to, sadly, powerfully reinforce age-old stereotypes.

I spent a couple of years working with the brilliant Jenni Regan and the media advisory service at Mind providing feedback on TV and film scripts that contained mental health storylines or references. One of my projects was a long-term *Coronation Street* storyline. The long-running British soap wanted to explore psychosis in one of its much-loved characters, Carla Connor.

I remember thinking how refreshing it all was because the *Coronation Street* team didn't use the go-to diagnosis of schizophrenia as a cause for their character's psychosis. Nor did they decide to bring in a new character who was "ready-made" with psychosis. If that had been the case, we'd have seen the illness before the person, which is never a good thing.

In choosing Carla Connor, a much-loved and well-recognized soap character, through which to explore psychosis, we were never going to see anyone other than Carla Connor, regardless of the symptoms she was experiencing. We already knew and understood her.

The fact that they chose significant stress and lack of sleep, alongside past mental health problems including additional trauma (baby loss) and depression, meant we were also able to separate out psychosis from schizophrenia and see that it can exist outside of that diagnosis.

The script team and the cast worked hard to consult with Mind's media advisory team and its information and legal teams, as well as experts by experience, ensuring that the result was accurate and de-stigmatizing. Because of this we saw the *true* vulnerability that psychosis creates in the person experiencing it.

Carla Connor is a formidable character – highly assertive, successful, sometimes ruthless and never one to take any shit. Experiencing psychosis did not make her violent or dangerous; what it did do is make her more vulnerable. She became confused and frightened. She needed help. But what was also refreshing was her recovery. The script team showed that recovery from psychosis is indeed possible and, although while symptomatic our personality traits (e.g. assertiveness, strength, resilience) can take a battering, we can regain them and recover. We can be the person we always were.

Indeed, there have been more positive portrayals of illnesses such as schizophrenia in the movies as well. *A Beautiful Mind* is one, although it really should be accurate given that it was based on the real life of a gifted mathematician!

Homeland is another more generally positive portrayal of mania and psychosis through its character, Carrie. It explores people's perceptions of her in terms of her ability to be able to do her job, and she ultimately proves them wrong. However, it also demonstrates how debilitating the illness can be and how some of the behaviours exhibited are incredibly problematic.

It comes back to nuance again. We feel for Carrie when people are undermining her, we worry about her when she is clearly unwell and we feel angry with her for behaving in some of the ways she behaves while unwell. It's not black and white. Mental illness – and life generally – never is.

the impact

I asked people how media portrayals in movies and on the news relating to their mental health problems impacted on their life.

"I first started hearing voices when I was a teenager. I went into hospital for a few weeks and when I came out I asked my best friend if I could stay at her house. Her mum said no. It turned out she'd seen a newspaper headline along the lines of 'Schizophrenic kills'. She thought that I might pick up a knife in the middle of the night and kill my friend's younger siblings or something. I lost that friendship forever."

"After I experienced postpartum psychosis, I felt as though people were wary of me. They were scared of the word psychosis, possibly automatically thinking the worst – rather than understanding that it is, in fact, a very treatable illness."

"It really frustrates me to hear the word 'psycho' being used. If only people knew what it actually was and that the vast majority of people experiencing it don't want to hurt anyone. I love a Hitchcock film as much as the next person, but the Psycho film created lots of enduring stereotypes with many people believing that, because of the title, the main character was psychotic."

"I went to a comedy night recently and the comedian was talking about her premenstrual dysphoric syndrome, a severe form of premenstrual syndrome. She went on to say that once a month she has a psychotic breakdown and turns into something out of The Exorcist. It was clearly a joke, but as someone who *has experienced psychosis I felt uncomfortable that the word 'psychotic' was being used to describe any manner of extreme behaviour as opposed to what it specifically is ... and how it was being conflated with 'being possessed by the devil'."*

This chapter is certainly not attempting to suggest that psychosis is a walk in the park and that there's no need to be afraid of it. It can sometimes be especially traumatizing for those experiencing it and their loved ones – just as any serious health problem can be. But what we mustn't forget is that those experiencing acute psychosis are more likely to be afraid of us than we should ever be of them. Much of our understanding of psychosis comes from portrayals in the popular media, portrayals that are all too often completely inaccurate. And this stigma influences how we behave toward people who may need our understanding, care and support.

The most important thing to take from this chapter is this: if somebody confides in you about their experience of psychosis, forget everything you *think* you know, and base your reaction on who they are as a person and what you see before your eyes. Horror movies and tabloid headlines give us nothing but sensationalism designed to draw us in and frighten us. Don't let them tell you what to think – see for yourself.

See the person, not the stereotype.

7

---

don't call me ... neurotic

Anxiety is one seriously broad topic. It is, after all, something that we all experience from time to time due to day-to-day pressures. Anxiety disorders, however, are something else entirely – they are relentless, overwhelming, often nonsensical, and can have a very real physical impact on us. The stigma comes from the lack of understanding about the difference between the two types, which might lead someone to downplay an anxiety disorder and ask the person, "What have you got to be anxious about?", inferring that they've got nothing to worry about and that they're overreacting. But, in reality, the thing they have to be anxious about is the anxiety disorder itself.

I know a fair bit about anxiety because I've experienced both types of anxiety since I was a kid. As an expert by experience, my understanding of anxiety versus an anxiety disorder is this:

- **Anxiety**: a response that is appropriate to the situation – for example, feeling anxious about a new job, moving house, having to give a presentation, being appraised at work, going on a first date, etc.

- **Anxiety disorder**: a disproportionate response to situations that may come on without any conscious train of thought. In my case, this has involved panic attacks about the bus I was travelling on randomly toppling over, panic about the cats being trapped in the dishwasher and panic about my throat spontaneously closing up.

Of course, the anxiety in an anxiety disorder can also relate to something that others are also anxious about (e.g. catching COVID), but the response is amplified and long-lasting.

Dr Stephanie de Giorgio, a GP, explains the difference from a professional's point of view. She said: "I would diagnose an anxiety disorder when the symptoms are persistent. So, although they might be triggered by an event, it persists past that for some time. Alternatively, I might diagnose an anxiety disorder if there is no real trigger for the anxiety. As a doctor I take a view on how prevalent and pervasive the anxiety is in the life of the patient, and how difficult it is making things for them. Obviously, there are DSM (*Diagnostic Statistical Manual*) criteria, but we don't really use those in primary care (day-to-day healthcare) – it's more about the impact on the patient's life."

The NHS website details different types of anxiety disorder and, as I have discovered, some can be experienced simultaneously:

- **Generalized Anxiety Disorder (GAD)**: a long-term condition that can make you feel anxious about a wide range of situations and issues.
- **Panic disorder**: a condition that causes recurring, regular panic attacks.
- **Phobia**: an extreme or irrational fear of something, like an animal or a place.
- **Agoraphobia**: several phobias related to situations such as leaving home, being in crowds or travelling alone due to a fear of being unable to escape a situation or being unable to find help if something went wrong.
- **Obsessive Compulsive Disorder (OCD)**: a condition that usually involves unwanted thoughts or urges, and repetitive behaviours.
- **Post-Traumatic Stress Disorder (PTSD)**: a condition caused by a frightening or distressing event.

There is also health anxiety, sometimes known as hypochondria, where a person has irrational obsessions about their health and a compulsion to Google conditions and seek reassurance from their doctor.

Dr de Giorgio told me: "Health anxiety is likely to be a sub-form of GAD, where the patient focuses on health. OCD and health anxiety can co-exist and also mimic each other, but OCD usually has the compulsive behaviours attached and health anxiety doesn't always have that. However, there may be OCD that is very much health-based. I usually first start to wonder about health anxiety if I see a person for the same reason a few times, and nothing seems to reassure them, including normal test results or examination. Or if they come to me repeatedly for different things and I am unable to link them together. It is important, of course, to ensure that there is no other cause of the symptoms and not to make the patient feel dismissed or that they aren't being taken seriously.

There are too many people, especially women, diagnosed with health anxiety when they have something physically wrong, so it has to be a diagnosis of exclusion. If health anxiety is diagnosed, we can begin to explain the symptoms and work on the issue."

As well as the panic attacks I've mentioned, which are more or less under control these days, aside from the odd occasion, I've been diagnosed with GAD and health anxiety over the years. Based on my own experiences, I totally agree that the key to understanding an anxiety disorder is understanding the level of distress it causes. For example, I have a phobia of spiders, but because I don't live in a spider- infested home the impact on my life is minimal. However, when I was younger, I experienced regular panic attacks that seemed to occur out of the blue, and some of which felt as though they lasted for around a week at a time. That was incredibly distressing and caused significant disruption to my life, as I was unable to enjoy myself, focus on anything else, concentrate on work, etc. I also had overwhelming thoughts of death that I was living with 24/7 during said panic attacks.

So, in this chapter I'm going to look at a couple of different stereotypes and misunderstandings that create the stigma around anxiety disorders.

stereotype: they're just being a hypochondriac

How many times have we heard – or even said – that phrase? I know I've said it about myself. I've made numerous apologies to family, friends, colleagues and, most significantly, my various GPs over the years for "just being a hypochondriac". The thing is, if you really *are* a hypochondriac in the true sense of the word, there's no "just" about it.

I want to explore why we are so dismissive of the idea of "hypochondria" and why we assume it means there is nothing wrong. There *is* something wrong. It's just that it's not the thing we *believe* to be wrong.

I also want to say to anyone who is struggling with health anxiety that you absolutely *can* recover. Sure, you might always be more vulnerable to health anxiety – or anxiety generally – but those periods of acute panic can't last forever. And the more you learn about it, the more you understand that you *do* deserve support (because you're not "just a hypochondriac" actually), and the more you reach out for it, the less frequent and less intense your anxious phases will become.

The impact of health anxiety on a person's life can be incredibly varied, as Dr de Giorgio has seen. "People might attend hospital or their GP surgery or call an ambulance multiple times a week. They might be unable to keep a job or manage a normal life because their anxiety consumes them. For others it will be less severe and they can function, but they will be anxious about symptoms and spend a lot of time on Google, etc. But I have had patients recover very well and find new ways of managing their anxiety in order to live a more fulfilling life."

here's my story …

Public health campaigns, such as ads on the back of buses about throat cancer and TV ads that help people recognize the first signs of a stroke, are great at raising awareness. They're designed to help people make better judgements about risks, and to seek help earlier rather than later. For most people, this knowledge enables them to act more quickly and limit the damage. For me, however, it can trigger a different kind of illness altogether …

As a teenager in the 1990s, with a steady boyfriend and a desire to be a bona fide grown-up, I saw my doctor and asked to be prescribed the combined contraceptive pill. I skipped home feeling like I was one step closer to realizing my dream of womanhood – one step closer to my idols who were totally already doing it. My teenage punk rock idols, Courtney Love and Kat Bjelland, were clearly already having sex. They were real women, who had sex, smoked and drank. And I was learning how to follow in their footsteps, albeit striking more of a Bambi on ice pose than fully fledged rock queen.

Growing up is awkward and, when you're prone to anxiety, the guilt you feel for doing all the things you're probably not mature enough to do intensifies. I was smoking Marlboro Reds, I was drinking Diamond White and I was *whispers* having sex.

Now all this guilt and anxiety didn't lay itself bare into some kind of easy-to- follow narrative. It wasn't dissected alongside *To Kill A Mocking Bird* in English Literature classes. It was lurking in my brain and my gut, but I had no real understanding of its presence.

Then one day, after a night at my boyfriend's bedsit in Hull, I noticed a mark on my arm. A tiny, freckle-sized blemish. The lurking guilt and anxiety immediately sprung into action, cross-referenced itself with the latest public health scare (the pill causes blood clots) and I immediately concluded that I WAS GOING TO DIE.

But this wasn't just a thought or a simple, fleeting worry. It wasn't a rational, OMG I'm going to fail my English exam because I wasn't *really* paying attention to what Atticus Finch was trying to teach his children. Of course I wasn't. I was discussing going on the pill with my best mate and covertly lending the cool girl a cigarette from my rarely used scrumpled-up packet of ciggies that I kept hidden in the bottom of my Head sports bag …

No, this wasn't just a thought or a worry. This was my first ever panic attack. And it went something like this …

I've got DVT. Shit. I've actually got DVT. I'm going to die. Like they said in the ads. Shit, shit, shit. I can't breathe. I feel faint. My heart is racing. Sweating ... Shit, I'm going to puke. I can't see anything. Hang onto the railings. Get to the pay phone. Call your mum. You need help NOW.

After much retching and half-walking, half-crawling along a busy shopping street in Hull, I reached the pay phone and spoke to my mum. She reassured me that a blood clot wouldn't look like a blemish on my arm. Perhaps I'd nipped my skin? She was right. My brain started to slow down. I wasn't going to die.

Unfortunately, the adrenaline was still pumping through my body. I walked back to my boyfriend's bedsit, still retching, still feeling faint, and sat on the cold concrete to bring myself round.

Eventually, the panic left me. But it came back. Again, and again, and again ...

If you had symptoms of feeling faint, having blurry vision, feeling nauseous, sweating too much and heart palpitations, you'd have good cause to see a doctor wouldn't you? However, as this merry-go-round blighted otherwise happy days (who am I kidding, I was a teenager, the days were probably already full of angst), I eventually went to see the doctor because I needed to check that I didn't have DVT, that my throat wasn't closing up, that my heart was normal and that I didn't have cancer (it's your glands, dear).

I had symptoms, but I was focusing on the wrong ones. I was diagnosing myself with an illness, but I was coming to the wrong conclusion. I had an illness. It was called health anxiety (later diagnosed as Generalized Anxiety Disorder because, well, my anxiety wasn't that fussy in the end).

As I discovered, health anxiety is an illness in its own right that causes all manner of problems and can take control of your life. The physical problems I've already mentioned are bad enough (and they're only the tip of the iceberg – you might also be sick, have diarrhoea, experience chest pains). But health anxiety affects your behaviours too – compulsive checking, prodding, picking ... I was always taking my pulse, checking my body for lumps, looking at my throat in the mirror to check it wasn't getting tighter. I didn't like taking tablets in case they got stuck, and I didn't like hot drinks because they made me more aware of the sensations in my throat.

Oh, but there was worse to come ...

Somebody invented Google. Well, that was me lost down a rabbit hole day and night – diagnosing myself with meningitis, cancer, heart disease, AIDS, Motor Neurone Disease ... you name it, I had it. And if there was a public health campaign, well, I didn't even have time to think it through before the familiar faintness and nausea washed over me.

The problem was, back in the 1990s, we didn't really talk about mental health. I had no idea I had a mental health problem. I mean, I knew I had these so-called panic attacks, but I was still convinced they were related to a heart problem or a blood problem or something. I didn't imagine for a second that they might be related to my brain. Brains are clever – why would it be the one part of my body that was messing up all the time?

I was offered beta-blockers, but I was scared of tablets. I think there was some talk of antidepressants too ... But eventually I was offered therapy and I sat and cried when it was offered to me because deep down, I knew I needed this help. I knew I needed to understand how to manage – and live with – the anxiety that plagued me.

stereotype: they're *so* OCD

There's been a long and stigmatized association of Obsessive Compulsive Disorder (OCD) and "being mega clean and tidy like Monica from *Friends*". People who love a neat minimalist home will sometimes describe themselves as "so OCD". This is problematic for those who do actually *have* OCD because, as they will tell you, it's not a choice.

Having OCD isn't about colour co-ordinating your bookshelves or neatly lining up your baked bean tins because you like the look of an orderly food cupboard. It's a distressing illness that can have a significantly detrimental impact on people's lives.

According to the charity OCD Action: "OCD is a clinically recognized disorder which affects around 1–2 per cent of the population. It is debilitating and paralyzing. People with OCD experience intensely negative, repetitive and intrusive thoughts, combined with a chronic feeling of doubt or danger (obsessions). In order to quell the thought or quieten the anxiety, they will often repeat an action, again and again (compulsions)."

Mental health nurse, Cara Lisette, has worked with many people experiencing OCD. She explains that it is an illness comprising intrusive thoughts and consequent behaviours that arise as a result of those thoughts. Cara said that, typically, when people think about OCD they might think of somebody having thoughts that they are going to become unwell as a result of contamination, so they might wash their hands frequently. She said that, while this is indeed representative of some people's experiences, OCD can present in many different forms and is a complex and debilitating illness.

Cara said: "There are different types of intrusive thoughts somebody might experience, including worrying that harm is going to come to them or somebody else, or that they themselves are a danger to other people and have, or are going to, hurt somebody. What is very important to recognize is that somebody having these thoughts in the context of OCD does not make them any more of a risk to other people, and they are likely to find these thoughts incredibly distressing.

"Due to the distress caused by these thoughts, people then start using compulsions as a way to neutralize them. These compulsions can be physical, such as touching things in a certain order, hand washing, putting things in particular places or following set routines; or mental, such as counting or repeating certain phrases in their heads.

However, there are many different compulsions somebody might be seen to be doing and this list is not exhaustive.

"OCD becomes very distressing and debilitating as people get stuck in a vicious cycle of completing compulsions to reduce the intrusive thoughts. However, this actually increases the intensity of the thoughts in the long run, resulting in more frequent or elaborate compulsions.

"Although OCD is very challenging to live with, it's important to recognize that, with the right treatment and support, a full recovery is possible."

stereotype:
PTSD – just a soldier's problem?

We often associate Post-Traumatic Stress Disorder (PTSD) with army veterans and, indeed, there are many who, after challenging and unimaginable experiences on the front line, do experience debilitating episodes of this condition. However, PTSD isn't something that *exclusively* happens to soldiers, and there are, in fact, many different ways in which somebody might develop it.

Ruth Cooper-Dickson, a trauma-informed coach, has worked extensively in this area. She says: "I've seen PTSD manifest in people who have suffered sexual abuse or domestic violence, or in those who have recovered from a significant illness. Refugees and displaced people might also experience PTSD, as might anyone who has been in a traffic accident, or been subject to a crime, for example. Put simply, PTSD can affect anyone who has experienced trauma. It becomes diagnosable as PTSD when the effects, which might include extreme anxiety, flashbacks, anger or lack of sleep to name but a few, are ongoing, significant and disruptive. For example, you wouldn't be diagnosed with PTSD 24 hours after the trauma occurred, but if you were still experiencing the symptoms several months later you might be. You can also experience secondary trauma, which is something we don't talk about as often. This is where you might witness a traumatic event that has happened to somebody else, for example, a fatal car accident. This can manifest as PTSD in some people, even though they didn't directly experience the accident themselves."

the impact

I asked people on social media to share their experiences of stigma relating to anxiety disorders. Here's what they said:

"People have said to me 'if you can talk to me you're obviously not experiencing a real panic attack. You're obviously doing it for attention.' It made me feel as though I had to make my symptoms even worse to be believed. To hyperventilate or shake more. And then of course that was followed by immediate thoughts of 'maybe I am faking it?'"

"My husband has OCD and I don't think people realize how bad it can be. Describing neatness as 'a bit OCD' is infuriating; it appropriates mental illness and creates an incredibly unhelpful public misunderstanding of the condition. I remember hearing a DJ say 'It would be great to have OCD as my house would be so clean,' completely misrepresenting a condition that has affected my husband's happiness all his adult life. Because of this minimizing of OCD, I think people are sometimes shocked or disapproving when my husband mentions he takes medication for it."

"When I disclosed that I had intrusive thoughts to my mental health service, they responded by threatening to call the police! It made me feel like I am a dangerous person and I couldn't speak about it again for years, which made my OCD even worse."

you can't "just stop it"

While knowledge is a good thing, and of course insight helps us to learn how to manage our symptoms, it doesn't automatically mean that we can "just stop" our anxiety symptoms.

Claire Eastham, a bestselling author, has written two books about her experiences of social anxiety and panic disorder. She says that, even though she now has an in-depth understanding of her condition, she knows that she can't simply tell her brain how it should and shouldn't behave. Claire said: "The amygdala is an aspect of the primitive brain and this can automatically override the rational. Basically, your amygdala doesn't give a shit what you know or whether you might make a tit out of yourself in front of Tom from HR or the woman at Tesco by "acting strangely". If it believes you are in danger, it will initiate the fight-or-flight response no matter how much logic you throw at it."

Claire had so many extreme panic attacks over the years that made her feel as if her heart was going to explode. She said "I had so many ECGs at the doctors when all the while my heart was perfect – it was my fucking brain that was the problem."

This is another area of anxiety that's interesting to note – the very real and physical impact that panic and anxiety can have on the body – shakes, sweats, dry mouth, palpitations, muscle tension, diarrhoea, vomiting … the brain is immensely powerful.

However, even though it sometimes feels as though her brain is beyond control, Claire still believes that knowledge can be really empowering. So, understanding your anxiety disorder and not being met with stigma is undoubtedly a huge help. And, as I've learned for myself, knowing that a panic attack is a panic attack and not, for example, a heart attack, can help to some degree. But because the experience in its own right can be so horrifying, the fear and anticipation that can build can create a vicious cycle.

This is why therapy and, in my experience, Cognitive Behavioural Therapy (CBT) particularly, can be so helpful for managing panic attacks. It's about teaching your brain tools and tricks and practising techniques to limit the force of the panic. For some people, including me, antidepressants or anxiolytics (anxiety medications) also help. Although they are not suited to everyone.

The brain is so complex and powerful, we'd surely have to be neuroscientists with super-powers to figure out how to "just stop" the panic and anxiety. But the more we learn, the more we can do to intervene and lessen the onset and severity of our panic attacks.

And if you're supporting somebody through a panic attack, acknowledge how frightening it can be, try distraction techniques, take part in breathing exercises, look at cat videos on TikTok but do not – under any circumstances – suggest that they need to "just calm down". It's really not that simple.

We don't need to be living in a war zone or a pandemic to feel overwhelmed by anxiety. The anxiety is based on, well, sometimes nothing, because it's an illness rather than a rational fear. But it still feels the same, and it can still be debilitating and, tragically, I have heard of people taking their own life because the distress of living with constant and relentless panic was too much to bear.

Anxiety disorders feel very future focused to me. We're not thinking about the now, we're thinking about *what might be*. And the *what might be* is usually catastrophic (in our own heads), which makes the panic and all the related physical symptoms ten times worse.

So, in response to questions such as "But what have you got to be anxious about?" I say this: "I don't know – it hasn't happened yet."

Anxiety disorders are very real. They are not merely a case of slightly increased exam stress or a bout of public speaking nerves. They can be debilitating, terrifying and overwhelming. And because these disorders are an illness, they have nothing to do with character or weakness. I've leapt out of a plane, abseiled into caves and spoken in front of hundreds of people at events. None of those things crippled me. Sometimes, however, with little warning, a very physical and frightening wave crashes over me and consumes me. And that certainly isn't because I'm frightened of the world. It's an illness. It's not me.

Anxiety disorders should be treated with the same respect as any other illness because, believe me, psychologically, it sometimes feels like you're battling your worst nightmare – times ten.

8

don't call me ... wino

Alcohol, drugs, sex, porn, gambling, shopping, gaming ... if anything's going to get your dopamine flowing, those words ought to do the trick. But not everybody uses these things for fun. Those of us who haven't experienced addiction have likely tried, and probably enjoyed, some of the drugs or activities that can lead to addiction, but we may find it difficult to comprehend how others react so differently to them. Why don't they just stop or enjoy them moderately, like we do?

Perhaps it's not so much about having a different reaction, as such, and more about having a very different need or reason for drinking or taking drugs, for example, in the first place ... perhaps a need to fit in, to be somebody else, to numb pain or to diffuse the impact of trauma.

"addicts brought it on themselves"

A piece of research I was involved with in 2019, while working with NewcastleGateshead Initiative and The Road to Recovery Trust, found that "1 in 3 people believe addicts brought it on themselves."

Dot Smith, CEO of Teesside-based charity Recovery Connections, is an expert in this area. She told me that it's the people struggling with addiction who probably feel that more than anyone: "The shame and distress brought on by living with the issue is enough on its own to perpetuate that mindset. While it's not for me to say that anyone is wrong in their own perception, based on their own experience, what I would suggest is that they ask another question – who would *want* to bring that on themselves?"

But is addiction ever a lifestyle choice? A bit of overexcitable partying that got out of hand? There's a big difference between getting off your tits on a Saturday night and needing to drink or use drugs, or do whatever you need to do, to get yourself safely through your day. Although "safely" is, of course, debatable given the huge number of alcohol- and drug-related deaths we see around the world. But for some people, it feels like the only option.

To anyone else, it seems crazy. Who would go to such extremes, using more and more of a drug (and I include alcohol when I'm talking about drugs – after all, it's probably one of the most dangerous), knowing full well that it could kill them? Or, if we think of addictions such as gambling or sex, knowing that it could destroy their life as they know it? Who would keep doing these same things over and over again, knowing all this?

They say that the definition of insanity is to keep doing the same thing and expecting a different result. But people struggling with addiction aren't really expecting a different result. As far as I understand it, they're more often than not unable to sit in their own skin and be comfortable. Or they're unable to relive their trauma.

Shahroo Izadi is a behaviour change specialist who has worked extensively in addiction and recovery. I asked her what she thought of the survey results that blamed people living with addiction. She said: "No one chooses to become addicted or wants to feel that they are at the mercy of a substance or behaviour that harms them and their loved ones and what they value most. An enormous amount of drug addiction can be traced back to trauma."

the role of trauma, pain and discomfort

The acknowledgement of trauma from Shahroo reminds me of an interesting podcast series – *Say Why to Drugs* – from researcher Dr Suzi Gage. Asking *why* the person is using the drug or participating in the behaviour is a much more impactful way to understand addiction. Shahroo said: "Far too often we focus on what is wrong with people's habits and why they don't change, despite knowing the negative outcomes and having all the resources, information and support available to them. Far more insight can be gained by shifting the focus to what someone is getting from a substance or unwanted behaviour in the moment. What purpose is it serving for them and when did that start?"

Indeed, Adam Ficek, psychotherapist, musician and drummer with Babyshambles agrees. He told me: "I view addiction as an attempt to fix something inside ourselves by using something outside ourselves. It's an attempt to self-soothe or regulate our emotions. At some point in our lives we have struggled internally and we find something that helps. We replay this again and again until the neuropathways become unconscious to an extent. This then forms into an unconscious behavioural pattern or addiction."

Adam admits that this is a generalized and simplified version of how he views addiction and that, in reality, it is far more nuanced, but it's a good starting point for those of us who haven't experienced the pull and desperation of addiction.

So, when we consider past trauma, perhaps drugs or behaviours are numbing or distracting the brain from reliving painful memories? Perhaps somebody feels so uncomfortable in their own skin that they can't function in the workplace or socially without masking who they really are and what they really went through? This then can affect people differently – as even when self-medicating (i.e. using drugs or alcohol to deal with a mental or physical health problem not otherwise prescribed by a medical professional), not everybody becomes addicted.

Blogger and author Claire Eastham lives with social anxiety and panic disorder. While she hasn't developed an addiction to alcohol, she has certainly used it to help her feel more comfortable. She said: "On the night of my second breakdown, I went to A&E with crippling muscle spasms in my jaw. After four hours of agony and having back-to-back panic attacks, I received only a 5mg tablet of Diazepam. It was a Friday night and, despite explaining that I wouldn't be able to see my doctor until Monday, they refused to give me an additional prescription. Bear in mind that this particular episode was so bad I had considered harming myself ... At 4am, back at home, I reached for the only option I had left – the one thing I knew would put my brain to sleep long enough to give me any respite ... alcohol. I drank half a bottle of rum straight (and I hate rum!) and I found it worked very quickly. It provided relief after hours of pain."

However, as Claire has discovered, alcohol takes as much as it gives. She added: "While alcohol takes the edge off when I'm in a state of panic, I have noticed that it makes my anxiety worse in the long run – particularly the following day. It makes me become more irritable and affects my sleep, so I try not to use it so much these days. In fact, during lockdown, I cut right down and I've definitely noticed a difference."

Hearing Claire's experience really reinforces the desperation involved in self-medicating. Claire used alcohol when she had nowhere else to turn, but then suffered the delayed consequences of using alcohol – while it may have helped in the immediacy, it created more anxiety the following day.

But, as Claire mentions, she has cut down. So why is it that some people can, whereas others can't? There isn't a simple answer to this, but it's clear that there are many contributing factors that cause the perfect storm for addiction.

Amy Dresner's story

Comedian and author of *My Fair Junkie*, Amy Dresner, grew up in Beverly Hills. She had a top-notch private school education and was a straight-A student. But she was also weirdly obsessive about purity and perfectionism. I spoke to Amy about her experience of addiction – something that left her with a permanent seizure disorder. She said: "It's ironic that I was so weirdly obsessive about purity and then went so far the other way, but that type of extremism is kind of classic for people with addiction." Amy struggled with depression as a teenager, suffered her first nervous breakdown aged 19 and another one aged 22. When she was aged 24 she discovered crystal meth. She said: "It seemed to help me manage my depression, numbing out the pain and the issues that I wasn't ready to deal with. As long as I was 'sick' and battling mental illness and addiction, I was able to dodge any real responsibility or focus on growing up or building a life. This was until, of course, it became a huge problem in terms of dependency, illegal activity, coming down, health issues, etc."

The impact that meth had on Amy was enormous. She was getting fired from jobs for drinking and drug use and was never functional while using. She also developed physical health problems, such as repeated infections in her nose and face. She said: "That's when I realized it was a problem and a prison."

Amy's appetite for meth use was so intense that even the other meth users she was living with in San Francisco would often comment on how concerned they were about her. This shows that substance use affects people differently – whether that's because of the problem driving the need, biology/genes, who knows. But one thing's for sure, when it came to Amy's drug use, she couldn't simply stop – even though she was struggling to function on any level and seeing her physical health decline as quickly as her mental health had. She added: "It was never a choice. It was an experiment that became a coping mechanism that became a terrifying compulsion. It would then morph to me abusing anything that would give me dopamine: coke, sex, shopping. The first time I did meth it was like a vortex opened inside of me. I had never experienced anything like it. Other people could take it or leave it and I was baffled by that. That's how I knew there had to be some weird biological component to it. Nobody wants to be an addict. And you don't know if you will be until it's too late."

addiction or dependency?

There is certainly widespread confusion around what it means to be "addicted" and what it means to be "dependent". And there is also a big difference between getting clean and sober and staying clean and sober.

The Surgeon General's Report on Alcohol, Drugs and Health: "Facing Addiction in America" talks about how scientific breakthroughs have changed our understanding of substance use disorders. It states: "Severe substance use disorders, commonly called addictions, were once viewed largely as a moral failing or character flaw, but are now understood to be chronic illnesses characterized by clinically significant impairments in health, social function and voluntary control over substance use." It goes on to compare addiction with some of the features involved in disorders such as diabetes, asthma and hypertension, stating: "All of these disorders are chronic, subject to relapse and influenced by genetic, developmental, behavioural, social and environmental factors. In all of these disorders, affected individuals may have difficulty in complying with the prescribed treatment."

Indeed, the first key finding listed in the report says: "Well-supported scientific evidence shows that addiction to alcohol or drugs is a chronic brain disease that has potential for recurrence and recovery."

The report talks about disruptions in three areas of the brain, including the basal ganglia, the extended amygdala and the prefrontal cortex. With those complexities in mind, it makes it perhaps a little easier to understand that telling someone to "just stop" isn't going to be fruitful. In fact, there are both physical and psychological factors in play that, unless we've been there ourselves, are nigh on impossible for us to comprehend.

I asked the experts how they would describe addiction and dependency in their words:

Shahroo Izadi said: "When it comes to alcohol, a lot of us would consider ourselves dependent: whether it's a dependency on it to make us feel more comfortable meeting new people or to destress after a difficult day. Definitions of addictions vary and, of course, physical addiction is a consideration in itself, but ultimately, if you feel that you're wanting to stop but you are unable to, then it's worth having a look at your behaviours and seeking support somewhere you can be totally honest without fear of judgement."

Adam Ficek said: "I view dependency through the lens of a physical dependency versus the behavioural and psychological process of addiction. Underpinning both these factors is the biological process of affect regulation, but in general, dependency could be, for example, where a 'heavy' alcoholic is only physically dependent and is able to withdraw effectively with a pharmaceutical intervention. This is different to the psychological and emotional distress of withdrawing from other process or substance addictions."

Amy Dresner said: "When you look at the science, chronic drug use actually changes your brain and creates both physical and mental dependency. It shuts down the brake system of the prefrontal cortex and you really don't have a choice. That part of your brain that regulates impulsivity, emotional reactivity and choice, is essentially hijacked. Eventually you can create new neural pathways but it doesn't happen overnight. It is also believed that there is a genetic component that interrupts your dopamine levels. Not everybody buys into the theory behind this but it makes sense to me as my mother and uncle were also addicts. But one thing that is absolutely key is that you must treat your underlying mental illness and trauma, otherwise it's close to impossible to stay sober for any length of time."

Dot Smith said: "Being addicted to a substance on *both* a mental and physical level causes tangible discomfort, and noticeable withdrawal symptoms. While the inability to obtain a substance someone is dependent on may be uncomfortable, and certainly occupy their thoughts, there's not the same level of obsession and desperation to get it as there would be if they were addicted. Plus, once a person is addicted, the idea of stopping becomes utterly terrifying. Imagine a train hurtling toward you and trying *not* to jump out of the way. It's that level of fear."

Again, what we need to look at is the *need*, not simply the behaviour. If the person was just drinking so much they became physically dependent, stopping might require a simple medical approach. However, and probably in most cases where somebody is physically dependent, where there was a psychological need in the first instance, a psychological and perhaps a social support approach may be needed to sustain that sobriety in the longer term.

Dot added: "If somebody was able to just stop, and they were able to get past any physical withdrawal symptoms, they may find they are left with aspects of life that they struggled to deal with before, and perhaps new problems that have been created during their substance use. Dealing with this, without the appropriate support, including the support of others who have been through what they have, is extremely unmanageable. This is something that is paramount in recovery – being able to see it in others and learn from their experiences is crucial."

a rock 'n' roll lifestyle?

I've always been interested in punk rock music and even wrote a novel in 2021, *The Twenty Seven Club*, exploring how we view musicians – especially rock musicians – who struggle with drug or alcohol use. It's easy to glamorize artists who use to excess, but when that goes beyond our appetite for rebellion, we shun them – or at the very least start to view them as unsavoury or bad ... The name of my novel is based on the media narrative about rock stars dying aged 27, which started to become popular following the death of Kurt Cobain. Other musicians who lost their lives at this age include Jimi Hendrix, Janis Joplin, Kristen Pfaff, Jim Morrison, Brian Jones and Amy Winehouse.

It's easy to be swept away by the wild behaviour we can find so appealing in our stars – and in the narratives the media spins. But when it gets too difficult, we can hold them at arm's length. We don't have to delve into their reality because they are not our loved ones. It's more difficult to see the truth behind the headlines.

I spoke to US writer and former musician Maureen Herman, who was one third of one of my all-time favourite punk rock bands of the 1990s, Babes in Toyland. Maureen told me that, due to the very nature of a rock show being at a bar or club, musicians are around alcohol and by association drugs every night that they are working. She said: "You're exposed to a lot of what would normally be social drinking, but it's a lot, because most social drinkers aren't at a bar every single night. So, it becomes difficult to separate what's normal and what isn't."

Maureen had no idea that she had a problem with alcohol while touring with Babes in Toyland, and it was only after she played Lollapalooza that the reality of her drink problem started to come to light. She said: "Of course, there were some problematic instances during the tour, but I first noticed that I was craving alcohol when I was no longer in that situation with others. When I was sitting at home and reaching for a drink each night."

Adam Ficek says that there is a combination of factors that make it difficult for some artists to thrive in the music industry. He said: "The combination of drug and alcohol accessibility, the pressure to perform, late nights and a lack of financial stability all contribute to the overwhelm of the music industry. As a musician and psychotherapist, I often feel that music and the music industry are two very contrasting and conflicting disciplines."

Although the perception of the rock 'n' roll lifestyle might be where we believe that a musician's problems begin, it's likely that the root cause began much earlier or, in some instances, later. Maureen said: "I was abused as a child, and, when I was touring, I struggled with major depression. However, it wasn't talked about so much then so I self-medicated with alcohol and cocaine. It was the only way to keep me playing and, on reflection, being in Babes in Toyland was one of the happier times in my life."

After Maureen left the band she was subjected to more pain and trauma when she was raped. She also lost one of her healthier coping mechanisms – her creative outlet and expression through music. It was at this point when things started to become unmanageable. She said: "When I stopped being in a band things got bad. The normalcy of being around alcohol was removed and I was left alone with an addiction. Things started to come to a head when I was fired from my job as an editor at *Musician* magazine because I couldn't handle my hangovers and kept calling in sick. This was the first time I sought treatment."

On reflection, Maureen, who is now 18 years clean and sober, completely understands the role that alcohol and drugs had in her life. She said: "It was a really great source of relief for me. Alcohol gave me a feeling of content and it eased a lot of my anxiety. It worked very, very well – up until a point when the consequences of drinking started to outweigh the benefits."

Maureen describes the tipping point as when the brain's primal reward system is set off and the urge to drink or do drugs becomes as strong as the instinct to run away from a lion. In effect, it is a compulsion to run away from and escape pain. She said: "A psychiatrist once told me I was seeking the same effect with crack that I would be getting with antidepressants – it was just that it was happening in a sudden spike rather than gradually over a long period of time." This is obviously why self-medicating becomes problematic – the effects are far more than therapeutic. However, Maureen believes that, given she had no understanding of depression, the effects of trauma and the treatments available, that if she hadn't had the accessibility and normalcy of alcohol and drug use, she might not have made it through those years. She added: "I knew that whatever I was getting from alcohol and cocaine was something that I needed. Rock n' roll provided me with that avenue and I don't know if I could have got through my 20s and 30s without it. I needed medication and this was the only way I knew how to get it."

a revolving door

If you speak to anyone who is in recovery from addiction, they will possibly say the same – that it saved them during a specific time in their life when they were struggling with something. But (and it's a big BUT) because of the nature of addiction, the substance then becomes the very thing that nearly kills them (or, tragically, does kill them in some cases) – or at the very least takes them to their rock bottom.

If this is the case, surely the answer isn't about simply stopping the drug or behaviour, but about dealing with the root cause as well? And this is where we become stuck in a vicious, revolving door cycle. A cycle that leaves the general public believing that addicts truly are hopeless ... Because the way many drug and alcohol services and mental health services are commissioned and designed separates the two issues. Often you can't see the crisis mental health team if you are intoxicated, but for those living with painful memories of trauma, significant self-esteem issues or other co-morbid mental health problems, the very idea of ripping open that wound by allowing the sober daylight to filter through is absolutely terrifying.

And perhaps that is why we see so many relapses. Because somebody might get detoxed in hospital then sent home – their physical dependency has been alleviated, but the root cause of their problem hasn't even been discussed. All too often, symptoms are being treated but the core problems are not.

And yet we still find it so easy to blame "the addict". They were given a chance and they blew it.

But what if you had pneumonia and pleurisy. You're given medicine to help you breathe more easily while you're all clogged up and your coughing is making you gasp for breath. You're given painkillers for the pleurisy that makes your ribs feel like they're ripping away from your lungs. But you don't stand a great chance of getting better if you don't treat the root cause – that pesky bacterial infection in the lung. You'll end up going back to the doctor or to A&E, and if they keep sending you home with painkillers and inhalers you may well end up just getting much worse.

Of course, there is a chance you might recover without antibiotics, but you're not being given the best opportunity. And it's the same with addiction – it needs a holistic approach because physical dependence is just one part of it. And from what I can gather from speaking to people who are in recovery, it's probably the quickest and easiest part of recovery to come to terms with.

substance hierarchies

I remember reading an article in the *Guardian* about how people dependent on prescription drugs should be offered separate rehabilitation. The article, which was published in November 2019, talked of how people dependent on prescribed opioids may feel uncomfortable seeking help from traditional "drug misuse treatment centres".

Maureen recognizes this hierarchy too. She said: "There is definitely a hierarchy of drugs and attitudes toward them. It's kind of like in school and there's the jocks and the popular kids and then there's the burnouts. And it's kind of like the alcoholics are acceptable, the cocaine addicts are kind of funny and daring but the heroin addicts are bad people. But we're all doing the same thing. We all have a different psychiatric need. But there was such a stigma around heroin. I shared it. I was like *at least I'm not doing heroin*. I felt superior. Heroin was for really bad fucked up people. It wasn't until later that I realized that everybody's drug of choice was basically a self-medication, they were choosing the regimen that worked for their bio-chemical make-up and what it lacked.

the impact of addiction stigma

The research shows that addiction stigma is rife, and I think we've probably all exhibited some level of it in our lives. I know I have. I remember when I was in my early 20s, saying to a friend: "Why do it? Life is good." I had no understanding whatsoever. I truly believed he could just quit, like it was a choice. Two decades later and, despite lots of episodes of physical ill health, he is still using. And while this type of stigma isn't something that is intentionally designed to hurt people (we sometimes say these things thinking we are helping), this lack of understanding can indeed cause harm. There's a saying: "secrets make you sick" – and this is so true in the context of addiction. Stigma pushes the problem underground where it becomes more isolating and far more dangerous. But in addition to that, it also creates wider mental health problems relating to shame, and it creates barriers to treatment, especially when health professionals use stigma. Amy Dresner said: "Even in recovery, I've had doctors who treated me differently or didn't believe I was sober because, as someone with a history of alcoholism, I wasn't to be trusted. I once had a stranger call me a 'crazy crackhead bitch' and I wasn't even using."

Amy also experienced stigma closer to home. She'd always been "the good girl" so when her father discovered she was addicted to crystal meth he was shocked and terrified. Amy said: "I had an infection at the time and was feeling really worried so I called my parents and my dad came to see me. He said 'You're a fucking drug addict. You're not my daughter. I don't know who you are, you're dirty.' Then he cried the entire drive back to Oregon. It was awful to hear those things, but I don't think he understood that at that point my addiction was a coping mechanism and a result of trauma and genetics."

Today, Amy's father, having seen the challenges she has faced and come out the other side from, has an entirely different view. Amy said: "When I got three years clean this time around I asked him if he was ashamed of me. He said, 'My friends wish they had a kid as unbreakable as you.' He now says I'm his hero and he totally appreciates and respects my resiliency."

---

the impact

I asked others to share their experiences of stigma relating to addiction. Here's what they said:

"I'd organized a business meeting with a highly recommended outside consultant, to discuss an upcoming project. While waiting for our visitor to arrive, my director whispered to me "Watch out, he's an alcoholic." I already knew this, however, and also knew how many years said "alcoholic" had been sober. "He'll probably have a glass of whisky under the table!", he added, joshing, before composing himself and returning to business mode. I worried what would happen if my old reputation ever came to the surface. Would I also be the butt of jokes in business meetings? And was I an alcoholic talented enough to keep on payroll? That important part of me, which I was usually comfortable sharing with people once I'd known them or worked with them long enough to build up trust, would have to stay buried here."

"The only people I would tell about my recovery journey are those struggling with addiction themselves and I thought I could help. Recovery has given me the understanding that I'm not other people's opinion of me. I don't need to share everything with everyone. Pre recovery, I was desperate for people's validation. I'm private about recovery not out of embarrassment or shame, I'm so proud of this journey. I don't share because I accept that often the world doesn't understand addiction and recovery, and I don't need to be judged by others to live a happy and healthy life."

"I was given an ultimatum by the Trustees of a successful eating disorders charity I'd founded. This came following a relapse from alcohol addiction and awaiting a second stint in detox and rehab. Clearly, my relapse was seen as a problem for a charity that worried more about its reputation than the wellbeing of its staff and volunteers. Rather naively, I believed I could be open about my current issues with alcohol in the same way I'd been open about my recovery from an eating disorder. I've often wondered if I'd relapsed to my bulimia (i.e. not alcohol), I might have been treated more fairly."

"What I found is that people's attitudes toward addiction is that "you've only got yourself to blame" and "you brought it on yourself – or, in other words, it's entirely self-inflicted. It seems people's ability to be empathic and compassionate is suspended when it comes to addiction."

"I had to write a formal complaint to the hospital trust that treated my daughter, who at the time was struggling with alcoholism but is now in recovery. The night shift healthcare assistant didn't give my daughter the help she needed. She had asked for a pillow because she was to remain in the reclining chair overnight and due to her being so underweight, her bones were protruding, making it really uncomfortable. The pillow never materialized. She also had questions about her medication, but every time she asked, the assistant spoke to her in a rude, offhand manner, or didn't bother responding to her questions at all. The next morning my daughter overheard her say to another member of staff 'that's her', at which point they both stared in her direction. Because of this, and the lack of support during the night, my daughter came to the conclusion that she was treated in this way because she was an alcoholic. Staff members should not discriminate between what they deem acceptable and unacceptable illnesses."

"I remember watching a comedian compare a struggle with addiction to that of battling cancer, ridiculing the idea and making fun of the institutions that are set up to help. I've since *understood that this was never the intention and that he was using comic effect to tackle a sensitive subject, however at the time this served to draw me further into my shell as someone not worthy of being helped. As a result I began to notice this attitude more and more in pop culture, certainly on the stand-up circuit, and even in sobriety I find it hard to watch this type of content as it engenders those shameful feelings of old."*

how can we change things?

As addiction is such a complex problem and, as Amy told me, 80 per cent of people who suffer have a comorbid mental health problem to add to the mix – it isn't as simple as "just stopping". Even if someone is forced to "just stop" it doesn't solve the root cause of the problem, and in some cases (particularly when it comes to alcohol), unsupported withdrawal can be incredibly dangerous.

But even if people are lucky enough to be surrounded by care, understanding and support, access to specialist services can be problematic. And I believe stigma plays a role here too, because those in charge of public funding may feel reluctant to invest in services that don't prove popular with the general public, a general public who don't understand the realities of addiction …

It's a vicious circle and I certainly don't have the answers, but I hope that in chipping away at stigma we can start to do *something* positive. If enough of us want to see people get well, maybe there will be more services funded in the future. I certainly hope so – far too many people lose their lives because of this cruel illness.

But, finally, I want to celebrate the strength and hope that can be found in recovery. I want to celebrate the people who have been caught in the depths of addiction and have managed to claw their way back out. As Dot said earlier in the chapter, "Imagine a train hurtling toward you and trying not to jump out of the way." The terror that people are trying to suppress, whether it be pain or trauma, is something I really can't imagine. But it's very real because, if you think about it, *nobody would choose* to live a life addicted. So those who find recovery are truly amazing, awesome, strong and inspiring people.

We'll finish on some words from Amy for anybody reading this who might themselves be struggling. And, remember, it took Amy eight rehabs, four psychiatric ward admissions, three suicide attempts and, finally, a felony arrest before she genuinely found recovery. So, it absolutely can happen – you can find recovery.

Amy says: "It's not your fault you have this but it is your responsibility to get better … I relapsed for 18 years before I got sober and now I'm coming up on nine years of sobriety. Relapse itself can become an addictive cycle, and it's easy to lose faith in yourself when you keep dropping the ball. Find somebody who believes you can get better and use their belief to fuel you to continue. Get connected with a supportive recovery community. Learn from your relapses, but don't let them define you. They say that relapse isn't part of recovery but I completely disagree – very few people get sober on their first try. Celebrate the small wins. Don't get caught up in perfection. DO NOT GIVE UP. If I can get sober, Jesus, anybody can."

9

don't call me ... vain

According to Beat Eating Disorders, the UK's leading eating disorder charity, there are around 1.25 million people in the UK suffering from eating disorders – many are doing so in secret. It's a similar picture in Australia, with approximately 1 million living with an eating disorder in any given year according to The National Eating Disorders Collaboration (NEDC). In the US, according to Mental Health America, there are around 20 million women and 10 million men who suffer from a clinically significant eating disorder at some point in their life.

But while the name – eating disorder – infers that it is very much all about the food, it is important to note that it is a mental health problem. Eating disorders can sometimes be caused by past trauma, too, with restrictive eating, overeating or purging being a manifestation of another problem.

Weight is, of course, a common talking point. However, as many contributors to this chapter agree, whatever your scales say, your weight is more a *symptom* of the problem – it never tells the full story.

it's not a vanity project

The stigma around eating disorders is still hugely problematic, impacting people both in terms of the way society views their illness, as well as their access to treatment. This, in turn, creates self-stigma (where the person internalizes the stigma and directs it against themself), which is particularly dangerous for those with eating disorders.

Campaigner and author Hope Virgo, who speaks regularly in schools and in the media, comes across stigma a lot in her work. She says: "People often view eating disorders as a vanity project, a diet gone wrong or just some teenage phase that's normal and that you'll grow out of. Some even see it as a lifestyle choice. On top of this we are still living in a society where people think that to have an eating disorder you have to be a certain size."

Hope's final comment, relating to size, shows how many people still struggle to understand that an eating disorder is a mental health problem, and that, even before weight is dramatically affected, the person may be experiencing significant internal distress that needs attention and treatment.

When Hope was just 13 years old she suffered sexual abuse and, to cope with her ordeal, she began restricting her food. She said: "I was sitting with these feelings that there was something categorically wrong with me and I needed to change that. Not only did the eating disorder give me this real purpose and value, making me feel enough, it also numbed so many of my emotions and so many of the things I couldn't bear to think about."

Hope became acutely unwell and was admitted to a psychiatric hospital where she was treated for a year. However, even though the illness threatened her life, and even though this was known to services, when she suffered a relapse in 2016, she was unable to access help. She told me: "I tried to access treatment, but I wasn't able to because I was not underweight – even though I recognized the signs that I was slipping back into those dangerous thoughts and behaviours."

Cara Lisette, a mental health nurse, was a young teenager when she was diagnosed with anorexia nervosa and purging disorder, which she often transitioned between. She said: "I can't say for sure what triggered it, although I recall having body image issues from around the age of seven. I had some difficulties in my personal life that left me feeling out of control, and I am hugely perfectionistic and often anxious. I also have a family history of eating disorders so, for me, it was likely a combination of genetics, personality type and the stressors I was experiencing in my day-to-day life."

Cara has undergone various treatments with both inpatient and outpatient care, and has continued to struggle with frequent relapses into her 30s, although now feels that she is in the best position she's ever been in to sustain her recovery. When I asked Cara about eating disorder stigma, she echoed much of what Hope had said. She also added: "There is this idea that everyone with an eating disorder is underweight, but in reality it's only a very small percentage of people. It's widely considered that anorexia is the most common eating disorder, when actually it's the least common. There's also this perception that everybody with an eating disorder wants to be thin, and that they feel this way because of celebrity culture. Although there are pressures from the media to look a certain way, an eating disorder is a serious mental illness and nothing to do with vanity."

There is also an idea that eating disorders mostly affect young, middle-class, white females. However, just as with any mental illness, eating disorders do not discriminate. According to the Butterfly Foundation, the national charity for Australians impacted by eating disorders, such disorders can affect anyone and occur across all cultural and socio-economic backgrounds, all ages, and in both men and women. The website states that males make up approximately 25 per cent of people with anorexia nervosa or bulimia nervosa and 40 per cent of people with binge eating disorder. In a recent study, lifetime prevalence for anorexia nervosa in adolescents aged between 13–18 years found no difference between males and females.

Underpinning Hope and Cara's experiences and knowledge, the Butterfly Foundation states that eating disorders come in all shapes and sizes and that "you can be considered a normal size" and "still have a diagnosis of an eating disorder".

In addition to the barriers to treatment, which may be caused by poor policies or a lack of understanding among healthcare professionals, Cara says stigma can create significant problems for people with eating disorders. She said: "Stigma can prevent people from seeking help, because they might not recognize that they have an eating disorder due to the misconceptions and stereotypes. And often people feel a huge amount of shame about reaching out for support when they don't feel that they are 'sick enough' to deserve it."

---

the impact

I asked people on social media to share their experiences of eating disorder stigma and how it impacted on their recovery. This is what they told me:

"In the UK, intense treatment is only offered when you are severely underweight, when in reality prevention of it getting to that point should be the key treatment. So many people try to seek treatment and are told 'you're a healthy weight' and it creates a belief in society that glamorizes thinness."

"The crisis team said to me 'we've never had a man before so we don't know what to do with you' followed by 'well something must have gone wrong when you were younger.' So there was the stigma that a) it's not a male illness and b) that it was somehow my family's fault. Another issue is that, although you hear lots about how women lose their periods, nobody ever really talks about the hormonal impacts on men and boys. My low testosterone went undiagnosed for years – my eating disorder had caused me to lose it."

"I often don't bother approaching medical professionals about my physical health issues as I know they will often just get blamed on my eating disorder and the risk of being triggered is simply too high. Eating disorders thrive off secrecy and stigma makes you want to keep your illness a secret so, basically, stigma is bloody exhausting and generally leads you into an endless cycle in which your eating disorder thrives."

"I've struggled massively with my weight and body issues my whole life. It took me a very long time to admit to myself that I had a problem, as it seemed like the sort of thing that teenage boys and young men don't get. I think there's still an unwillingness to discuss eating disorders in men – there's still a perception of them being the sole territory of young girls/ women. It all comes under the toxic masculinity umbrella, I think, the way these things aren't talked about. A lot of men have problems enough talking about their mental health as it is, but there's still a real stigma attached to eating disorders that makes them doubly hard to discuss."

tackling the stigma

As we have found time and again, stigma is a significant problem when it comes to providing the right services to the people who really need them. In 2018, Hope launched the "Dump the Scales" campaign to combat the issue of people being unable to access treatment because of their Body Mass Index (BMI). This clearly links to the stigma that eating disorders are all about weight. Hope's petition now has almost 120,000 signatures, and it has taken her to Downing Street to chat with UK members of parliament about the need to change the criteria around treatment admission. Hope added: "Not all eating disorders are visible. They are a mental illness and, just because somebody looks OK or has a so-called healthy BMI, it doesn't mean that they *are* OK."

As health professionals, friends, family or colleagues of somebody with an eating disorder, we need to remember that it isn't a "lifestyle choice" or a vanity project. Just as we shouldn't suggest that somebody with an addiction "just stops", we also shouldn't suggest, as Hope says, that someone with an eating disorder "just have a burger and fries". Eating disorders are very real, highly complex and incredibly dangerous mental health issues. Assumptions should never be made about why a person is experiencing this severe mental health problem because, as we can see from what people have told us from their own experiences, this can trigger even more devastating behaviours and problems. We should also remember to withhold any comments about how somebody looks on the outside. It might not match the turmoil that is taking place on the inside.

10

---

don't call me ... flawed

Imagine what it feels like when you're given a diagnosis of personality disorder. Our personality is who we are, and being told there is something wrong with it, that it is disordered in some way, must be quite earth-shattering. On the flip side, some people find labels and diagnoses useful – even the personality disorder ones – because it helps them understand more about why they have felt the way they have for so long. Either way, there is a huge lack of knowledge around personality disorders in terms of what they are and the different types.

This chapter isn't designed to argue for or against the use of personality disorder labels, but more to deepen our understanding of what those labels mean so that we can avoid using stigma.

- **Borderline Personality Disorder (BPD)**: also known as Emotionally Unstable Personality Disorder, BPD is described on Mind's website as having difficulties with how you think and feel about yourself and other people. There may be very significant worries about being abandoned by people, and emotions can be incredibly intense and change very quickly. There are often impulsive behaviours, self-harm and suicidal feelings. Some people also experience paranoia or dissociation.

- **Narcissistic Personality Disorder (NPD)**: according to Mind, people with NPD may believe they are special or more deserving than others but, conversely, they are likely to have fragile self-esteem (and therefore rely on others to recognize their worth). See also page 35.
- **Histrionic Personality Disorder (HPD)**: a condition in which people feel uncomfortable if they are not the centre of attention. They may feel that they need to entertain others and constantly seek approval. See also page 27.
- **Antisocial Personality Disorder**: when someone puts themself in dangerous or risky situations, behaving illegally, feeling easily bored, having problems with empathy and becoming aggressive. This is a fairly controversial diagnosis that some people relate to psychopathy (see also page 101).

These are just a small number of the different personality disorders that are listed in the DSM (*Diagnostic Statistical Manual*) and, as you can see, they describe very different traits. The stigma comes into play because the "personality disorder" label is consistently used across all of these diagnoses, making them often lumped together in our minds and causing the huge differences between the characteristics to be overlooked.

personality disorder diagnosis and identity

Both Dr Malkin and Dr Muñoz Centifanti, psychologists who we have met in previous chapters, have worked extensively with patients who have been diagnosed with personality disorders.

Dr Malkin said: "Personality disorders are all extreme versions of normal personality structure; that is, we used to routinely distinguish between, say, obsessive compulsive *character* and obsessive compulsive *character disorder*. The former may be a scientist who values the world of ideas, problem-solving and routine more than adventure, risk and emotional ecstasy; the latter is the person who so prioritizes an orderly environment and intricate thought over other approaches to life that they completely alienate their partners with their rigidity and aloofness. All personality disorders fall on a spectrum. Character/personality structure tells us a person's favoured way of approaching life and relationships, while character/personality disorder as a label indicates that the approach has become so rigid that the person struggles significantly both emotionally and psychologically."

Dr Muñoz Centifanti puts it this way: "All personality disorders are interpersonal. You can't have a paranoid person without considering their relationship with others – i.e. without them thinking that others are against them. Similarly, with BPD, it doesn't make any sense unless you're also thinking about how that person is feeling and responding within relationships i.e. thinking others might reject them. The relationship with others should be considered a key factor."

Of course, even within expert communities there are debates around the types of personality disorders and what they mean. Dr Muñoz Centifanti, for example, doesn't believe in the diagnosis of antisocial personality disorder, as she believes this doesn't fit with the interpersonal theme that runs through all other personality disorders. She said: "Antisocial personality disorder is more societal than interpersonal. It relates to how the individual behaves within societal norms or expectations, rather than relating to disruptions in personal relationships, although the diagnosis has changed over time."

This is where Dr Muñoz Centifanti feels that psychopathy has a role within personality disorder diagnoses. "Psychopathy is about people. It's interpersonal because it's about how the individual relates to others. For example, having a lack of empathy toward others and a lack of guilt or remorse are about feelings for other people's distress."

If we take Dr Muñoz Centifanti's understanding of personality disorders, then it's less about identity and more about how people have learned to respond, behave or feel in different contexts. The person diagnosed is separate from the personality disorder.

the stigma of personality disorders

It is helpful to explore *why* clinicians use labels for personality disorders. Dr Malkin said: "Recognizing that someone suffers from a personality or character disorder helps clinicians to restore flexibility and functioning so the patient can embrace the best that their personality has to offer. However, labels like personality disorder are *most* helpful when they're in the background, guiding us to understand what makes someone tick well enough to get all their psychological gears into working order. When they become the foreground to understanding *who* someone is, they collapse into stigmatizing slurs."

Something else that is clear from speaking to experts by profession and experts by experience is that there are different levels of stigma depending on which PD diagnosis you receive. I spoke to one woman who was diagnosed with both BPD and Anxious Avoidant Personality Disorder. She told me that she didn't feel as strongly about her diagnosis of Anxious Avoidant Personality Disorder because it isn't demonized in the same way as BPD.

She said: "I knew my anxiety was not normal and getting that diagnosis was, in many ways, validating, reassuring and comforting. People find anxiety easier to understand. The BPD diagnosis, however, felt like a punishment. It was as though I had a label placed on my forehead telling all professionals that there is something inherently wrong with my personality. It's been a barrier to treatment because I feel that most psychiatrists I've worked with were hesitant to hospitalize me when I really needed to be admitted. And nurses in A&E would say unhelpful things to me like, 'weren't you just here last night'. I also felt that duty CPNs (Community Psychiatric Nurses) would not come to see me because of how often I presented at crisis point. Why is that OK? A sore throat does not become any less sore just because you tend to get it a few times a month. And suicidality and other BPD symptoms do not get any less painful or challenging to go through just because they creep up so often."

Conversely, however, she did find *some* comfort from the label. She added: "In some ways the diagnosis was a relief because at least now I know why I am the way I am. At least it's a condition that I can look up, educate myself about and talk to others who also have the same diagnosis as me."

Dr Muñoz Centifanti agrees that labels have both positive and negative impacts. She added: "I'm not going to tell people what labels they can and can't have. I think a lot of people have these personality disorder labels but really, there's nothing wrong with the person (like the label implies), the problem lies with interpersonal problems – and I believe that interpersonal problems can be solved or at least managed."

the impact

I asked people on social media to share their experiences of personality disorder stigma and how it impacted them. This is what they told me:

"I am diagnosed with BPD but it took the professionals a long time to say it. My first therapist hid it from me, which I think she did to protect me. But when I found out I felt more confused. On a positive note, the diagnosis helped me to understand myself and my behaviours better. I found it comforting to understand why I did what I did. However, I do tend to hide behind my other diagnoses of depression and anxiety, because I feel worried about how people will react when they hear I have a personality disorder."

"When it comes to PDs I feel as though the most stigma comes not from society generally, but from within mental health services. If those trained in mental health have such attitudes, what hope is there for those who have no understanding in the first place. For me, personality disorder as a diagnosis – regardless of type – should be abolished. As long as the label exists, the stigma will remain. How can we say there is something wrong with someone's personality, that they are flawed, when personality is such a unique thing."

"My diagnosis made me feel like I wasn't capable of having a full life due to the connotations that come with BPD. But in the same breath it made me feel like there was a name for some of the problems I was having and that I wasn't a defunct human being. I had an illness and I could work on that. I have

only experienced a small amount of stigma as a result of my diagnosis but it is still damaging – the minimizing or dismissal of serious symptoms especially in relation to self-injury and suicidal behaviour. A staff member in A&E rolled her eyes at me during one admission."

"I was angry when I was given the BPD diagnosis. I was told that my rejection of it was a symptom of it, but the diagnosis caused so many problems for me. It led to the removal of my previous diagnosis of schizophrenia, which I believe I actually do have. And it also led to the removal of the support that I was accessing for schizophrenia. The stigma I have experienced has mainly been from within mental health services, where there is sometimes a culture or policy of not actively responding to the needs of a BPD patient (known as positive risk taking). This led to me being discharged when I was in the middle of a psychotic episode once."

"The diagnosis helped me piece together parts from my life experience that I hadn't previously understood. Although when I first got diagnosed, everything I did I put down to BPD. I actually wasn't aware of any stigma until I started more publicly sharing my own experiences. I once had a comment from a stranger saying that I deserved all the BPD stigma I got. And another person who automatically assumed I was controlling and abusive because of the BPD diagnosis."

---

stigma among mental health professionals

It is clear from talking to people diagnosed with a personality disorder that stigma can be an issue within mental health services. However, on speaking with Dr Helen Casey, a researcher who has spent many years facilitating group therapy with people diagnosed with a personality disorder, the reasons for this are a bit more complex than we might first imagine. It simply isn't just a case of the mental health professional not understanding what a personality disorder is, it's possibly more to do with the service structure and available treatment options that they are working within – and also what types of responses they are used to seeing.

Dr Casey told me: "In my experience, there is often a sense of hopelessness around BPD in mental health settings because general treatments are not all that effective. So it can seem, to the mental health professional, that somebody with BPD is untreatable. However, this is because the individual needs more specialist support. For example, mentalization-based treatments and schema therapy (a type of therapy with a strong emphasis on relationships) have both been shown to be effective in the treatment of BPD. You are less likely to find stigma in a specialist personality disorder unit or service for two possible reasons: firstly, the professional has chosen to help people with personality disorders specifically and secondly, because the treatments are designed specifically for such patients, and therefore are more likely to be effective.

"Additionally, there's a notion of the 'revolving door' for those diagnosed with BPD, where people can do really well for a long time and then suddenly relapse. Staff who are used to this presentation are more likely to see the bigger picture and the positive outcomes for the individual based on their period of being well, rather than seeing it as a failure in the treatment. They are therefore less likely to feel frustrated and display these feelings."

According to Dr Casey, research suggests a link between trauma and BPD, and many individuals diagnosed with BPD have experienced childhood trauma, sexual abuse and/or disorganized attachments (e.g. unhealthy or inconsistent relationships with parents/loved ones).

Dr Casey says that, as there are often traumatic factors involved, a trauma-informed approach that provides a new narrative may work well. She said: "A re-parenting approach can work well. What I mean by that is providing the individual with the kind of approach that they never had in childhood, and building on that as you would a child." Dr Casey is careful to stress that this doesn't mean treating the individual like a child, but more empowering them to trust and start to build their own narrative, one that helps them to feel more secure in terms of their attachments or relationships with others. This is often what was lacking in the person's original experience of being parented. She said: "This kind of work takes time, and that's OK. Off-the-shelf therapies that might last six or twelve sessions are not the best option in cases of BPD, and that's where some professionals may feel frustrated. This is probably seen as a more old-fashioned approach, but sometimes that's what is needed. Lots of patience and acceptance is key to helping the person to manage not only what their current symptoms are, but also how to thrive in the longer term."

This is the interesting thing about stigma – it is often driven into society by the way in which policies are written or services commissioned or funded. If people are in the wrong service, both the patient and the professional can feel frustrated. Of course, the impact on the patient is going to be paramount here (although not exclusively) and, as we know, often we are not dealing with model professionals – or indeed patients. People are people regardless of their role or diagnosis. But it's interesting to learn that, perhaps in many cases, the problem lies behind the scenes – in the budgets for specialist services, in the commissioning (or lack of) of these relevant services and in the training available to staff. After all, a patient with cancer will not do well on a stroke ward and vice versa, so why are so many people with personality disorders treated in general mental health settings?

but aren't *some* personality disorders inherently bad?

While people with BPD, for example, demonstrate often quite vulnerable traits and might often be at risk of suicide or self-harm, what about those less vulnerable people? What about psychopaths?

Surely this book isn't about to say that, actually, we've got it all wrong. Those murderers locked up in prison with zero empathy for anyone, they're people too, they have an illness too. They need our understanding and we shouldn't stigmatize them because of what we see in the movies?

Don't worry. I'm not about to argue that we should provide tea and sympathy for the devil! But, actually, while such individuals might *seem* like the devil incarnate to us, they were once born innocents. And although there are certainly people in this world who have grown and developed into dangerous individuals, who might no longer be suitable for rehabilitation or release, what if we met them decades earlier?

We hear many backstories of infamous killers being subject to trauma or abuse growing up. It's difficult to conjure sympathy for them when all we see is the face of the killer. But what if they were supported when they were children or young adults?

Dr Muñoz Centifanti works with children who have callous and emotional traits, and she is often ridiculed for suggesting that such children can and should be supported and rehabilitated. She said: "I get so many comments on my TED X talk about being stupid. Probably in some cases it's simply because I'm a woman, but it's also because I have seen evidence showing that parenting is a way to deal with callous and emotional traits. There's a view, one that I've even seen during peer review of my published findings, that you can't change these children and that we should lock them up from day one. But I truly don't believe that should be the case. I have evidence from dozens of studies that warm, firm and responsive parenting and rehabilitation work – although it's certainly challenging work. With the right, specialist kind of treatment there is hope, but it has to be the *right* treatment. And I think that, if we recognize the problem, not only can we affect change in the development of infants and toddlers, but also in adolescents too. No age is beyond help."

Dr Muñoz Centifanti explains this in terms of prison populations and how, just as people with specific mental health problems are often treated generically in society, so too are some individuals in the prison community. She said: "If you consider that more than 80–90 per cent of prison populations are made up of people who are much more impulsive and emotionally dys-regulated, and you decide there needs to be some sort of rehabilitation, you might bring in psychologists who look at the common themes. Lack of education, hot-headedness, for example. Programmes are built around these commonalities but the kind of treatment they offer will likely be ineffective for people with psychopathy. But we try to put them through the programme regardless, and then they come back with another crime, so we say, there's nothing that can be done for them. But the programme isn't being designed to treat psychopathy, it's designed to treat those other issues that they don't have as much. So, it's not going to work. It's like in the cartoon, *The Simpsons*, saying 'we've tried nothing and we're all out of ideas.'"

Dr Muñoz Centifanti explains that, in childhood, those growing up in abusive and traumatic environments (as many psychopaths do) might learn to shut off their emotions to enable them to recover more easily from the traumas they face. The more they do this, the more likely they are to get better at it. This can therefore develop into callousness or lack of empathy, as it becomes easier and easier to shut off emotions. She said: "Maybe a two-year-old learns how to recover emotionally from a knock because they've had to. By the time they're five, they might be breaking someone else's toys. By the time they're nine, they could be punching someone in the school yard and not feeling bad about it. We need to teach those children how to feel empathy and acceptance and self-compassion. They need to learn how to accept negative emotions. The earlier we get to work with these individuals the more hope there is. But we shouldn't consider all children and adolescents showing callousness as untreatable. They deserve a chance to recover."

stigma by association

It is the "personality disorder" part of the label that can put those with BPD under the same umbrella as those with psychopathic personality disorders and this creates stigma by association. Just as psychopathy and psychosis are pretty much polar opposites, sharing the first few letters in their names has created confusion among some of the general public. But sometimes it's better to address this directly. Call out the confusion and shine a light on the difference. Put the two opposites together to show the stark contrast. A primary colour stands out much more brightly when sitting next to a pastel hue.

From speaking to the experts, we can see that the "personality disorder" part of the diagnosis has *absolutely nothing* to do with *who* the person is or what their *personality* is *like*. It is more about recognizing that an individual needs longer-term and specialist care because their problems are more complex and have developed over a long period of time – often since childhood. It certainly doesn't mean people with personality disorders share the same behaviours or traits. For example, somebody with BPD might struggle with too much empathy for others, while someone with psychopathy might struggle with too little ...

It seems that we are absolutely right when we say that everyone's personality is unique – just like every snowflake! And just because you have a specific personality disorder label it doesn't mean that you are like anybody else with that specific label. People with BPD might share some of the same struggles as others diagnosed with BPD, but they are still individuals with unique personalities. You are no more or less likely to enjoy classical literature or celebrity gossip just because the next person with BPD does.

So never mind the gaps between the different personalities being so vast, we need to remember that even the *specific* personality disorder diagnoses do not have any bearing on *who* a person is. Only what they might *need*.

11

don't call me ... bad

We know that there's a significant lack of mental health services and that many people wait months – sometimes years – to access treatment. It's therefore unsurprising that sometimes people turn to unhealthy forms of self-medication such as drink or drugs. And such forms of self-medication can lead people into all kinds of trouble.

Mental health stigma may of course be one factor, whereby individuals might feel ashamed to speak out and seek help, or not have the understanding or knowledge to see what's going on and therefore seek the appropriate help. They might turn to coping mechanisms that temporarily relieve symptoms or pain in the short-term, but in the longer term create an avalanche of additional challenges, sometimes involving the law.

Of course, the majority of people with mental health problems don't end up in the criminal justice system, but of the people in the criminal justice system, many have experienced complex, disadvantaged backgrounds combined with mental ill health or psychological trauma.

There are many matters of psychological trauma that we might not see or know about when it comes to people who have offended. Are people being coerced and controlled by an abuser, for example? Are they forced to commit crimes? Are they scared of leaving an abuser for fear of retribution? Do they keep letting their abuser back into the home because they see it as the only way to survive? Trauma that is being experienced on a daily basis, and where the victim is unable to seek respite or psychological support, might create another route into the criminal justice system.

Education and background are other big factors, as many people in the prison system might be unable to adequately read or write due to a chaotic upbringing or undiagnosed developmental issues, which we know can also lead to mental health problems (according to a study cited on www.mentalhealth.org.uk, 54 per cent of people with a learning disability also have a mental health problem).

Research shows that around 70 per cent of people in prison have a mental health problem. But within the prison system, individuals often come from complex and chaotic backgrounds. So we can't suggest that poor mental health is either the main cause or the main outcome – there are so many factors that combine to create the perfect storm. But it is *definitely* there and definitely has a significant role to play. In the prison system, an individual's ongoing experience of stigma and discrimination is amplified enormously. You could say it's a spiral of stigma that becomes worse and worse the harder life becomes.

This is why I wanted to write this chapter. To stop and think – not just about the direct stigma of mental health problems, but about the stigma of the *consequences* of the mental health problems and psychological traumas that some people face.

We need to keep in mind that not everyone who experiences significant mental distress has been diagnosed with a specific illness. I think it's also important to recognize addiction as a mental health issue, (as well as a physical and social issue) – in addition to a coping mechanism or self-medication for mental health issues or mental health stressors (such as poverty or abuse).

Finding the beginning of the tangled thread might be challenging, but mental health is almost always wrapped up in it somewhere.

does every crime deserve punishment?

It's easy to assume that everyone who is "punished", for whatever reason, is deserving of such punishment. In some ways, perhaps it helps? Perhaps prison is the only place they can access mental health support? Maybe in some cases prison gets them away from abusive partners or associates? Sometimes, particularly when you look at the 12-steps to recovery from addiction, we can see that there is an onus on admitting "the exact nature of our wrongs" and making amends – something that forms a key part of recovery. But in the end, even though some people might benefit from accessing a rehab programme in prison, it's rarely the answer. And what if the crime is only committed in the first place as a cry for help?

If mental health services and interventions were sufficient (and mental health awareness more widespread and stigma less so), then many individuals may not need to go to prison to access treatment and would therefore transition into recovery without a criminal record tarnishing their lives. And if the prison system had more focus on rehabilitation, and less on punishment, perhaps the revolving door might stop revolving.

We shouldn't assume "badness" just because somebody has been sent to prison. We don't know their circumstances, and, upon release, "justice" has been served anyway. However, following release and longer term, there is likely to be stigma, shame and discrimination impacting their social lives, family life, housing situation and employability.

It's also interesting to question the system itself. Just because it *is* that way, doesn't mean it *should* be that way.

Centuries ago, you might be considered a "witch" if your punishment (drowning) didn't kill you. There was no way out of that one! We can challenge the way things were then, so perhaps we shouldn't automatically accept the system for how it is today, either? There was a time when people really did believe in those witch trials ...

But either way, these days, if you have a significant mental health problem and adopt an unhealthy coping mechanism that leads you astray (because it's the only way you know to survive), you can end up with the label of criminal ... and that's something that sticks around for a long time.

why do people end up in prison?

Richy Cunningham has 20 years' experience working across addiction and criminal justice services in the North East of England. Richy says that by the time most (almost all) people reach the criminal justice system they have been involved with (and therefore failed by) other parts of the health and social care system – be that an addiction, mental health or housing service, or at the very least they will have spoken to their doctor about substance use or mental health issues. He said: "This is in relation to people who were adults at the point of entry into the system, but those who entered as a young person will, more often than not, have been diagnosed with a mental health issue or have had an addiction issue as a child, which has continued into adulthood."

According to a 2021 evaluation into the Fulfilling Lives programme (which aims to support people with multiple complex needs), the researchers reported that multiple disadvantage "tends to be associated with persistent and low-level offending, such as shoplifting and theft, often driven by addiction." It also states that "short-sentence prisoners are often affected by homelessness, substance misuse, poverty and debt." Anything driven by addiction is driven by a mental health problem, as addiction, in my view, is a serious mental health issue often relating to trauma or co-morbid mental health diagnoses. But we also know that homelessness, poverty and debt all significantly impact mental wellbeing, and that even where addiction doesn't come into play, substance misuse can be part of a need to "self-medicate" or switch off from a chaotic and frightening environment. The report also refers to a 2018 Female Offender Strategy, which states that almost half of female prisoners say they committed their offence to support the drug use of someone else. Why might this be?

young offenders

Beverley Hunter, Research and Evaluation Communications Lead for Fulfilling Lives, told me that, when it comes to teenagers and young offenders, you will very often see that they fit a certain "model" – even though their experiences are unique, there are lots of similar themes. She said: "When you talk to them to find out why they offend, you'll find that there are themes such as undiagnosed neurodiversity, poor educational attainment, trauma, poverty, drug use and so on. Once they find themselves in the criminal justice system, a lot of young people struggle to escape from it. They don't know how to remove themselves from the people and the area that encourages these activities – and often it's within their families as well. So it's very difficult to get out of once you're in it."

Beverley explained that a lot of young offender crimes are drug related – selling drugs or thieving to pay for drugs – and that while there's a lot of addiction, much of it is down to recreational drug use. However, the kind of drug use she hears of from those coming into prison settings is very different from groups of partygoers taking drugs for a high or a new experience. She said: "The recreational drug issues we hear about in the prison system are far more problematic. This tends to be people wanting to get off their faces as quickly as possible. To block the world out and escape something. Many would seek the hardest drugs they could find to switch off from the world around them."

This is an example of how environmental/social stressors and trauma can lead to drug use. Dependency/addiction might not always be the end result, but the reason for using substances is to manage mental stress.

Beverley said: "I remember one story of a guy who was repeatedly overdosing on Valium, so much so that he had massive burns on his feet because he would fall into a deep sleep in front of the fire. And a lot of drug use in prison is far from fun. You'd have people getting incredibly ill from spice or from the methadone substitute, buprenorphine, also known as subutex or 'subbies', which, when crushed and snorted, would give people a very acute, intense high that lasted only briefly. Then they'd spend the rest of the evening struggling with vomiting and diarrhoea. You'd ask why they do it, because the effects looked absolutely horrific, but they would tell you it was worth it for that momentary buzz. That brief escape." Clearly, this is another form of self-medicating, to remove yourself from whatever mental distress your environment or past traumatic experiences have created.

This all relates to the conversations in chapter 8 (see page 137), where we try to understand *why* people take drugs in the first place. What are they trying to escape from or soothe? I think the subutex and spice examples say a lot about what people are dealing with in terms of their environment or their psychological state. It certainly isn't an all-night rave. It's more like an all-night sickness.

So, this type of drug use can lead people to prison *and* keep them coming back in later years. And it's likely to be driven by very difficult life circumstances that many of us are privileged enough not to be able to comprehend. Beverley added: "It sounds very clichéd talking about people coming from broken homes but it's true. You do an offender assessment when people come into the system and you absolutely will find those poor educational backgrounds, developmental issues, violent home lives and so much more. Again, people's choices are limited in ways you or I might not be able to understand."

women in prison

When it comes to women in prison, there are often different factors driving their incarceration. Beverley told me that this often relates to crimes of passion, for example, theft to feed the family, or violence against an abusive partner in retaliation. There might also be crimes that women are forced to commit by a partner. Again these issues relate to very challenging life circumstances, whether that be poor educational attainment for the reasons already discussed above, and therefore poor chances of employability, or coercive control and domestic violence. So mental distress and psychological trauma are again at play.

Open Clasp is a theatre company that has worked extensively with women affected by the criminal justice system in order to give them a voice and be heard. The company aims to raise awareness of the issues women face. In 2014, the company was commissioned to work on a new play, *Key Change*, aimed at giving a voice to women inside the prison service and exploring the routes to prison and the "why". The play became a huge hit, touring theatres and prisons in the UK and also in the US, where it received rave reviews on Broadway. It has also been performed at the Houses of Parliament to parliamentarians and policy makers, complete with a post-show talkback and Q&A with Baroness Corston – author of a report into vulnerable women in the prison system. The play was one of several contributing factors to a debate that led to the Prison Safety and Reform White Paper. Meanwhile, while the play was in New York, post-show discussions took place with international experts on the issues of women in the criminal justice system, including award-winning researchers Evan Stark and Professor Rosemary Barberet.

By working with women with lived experience, Open Clasp found that many women had experienced domestic abuse and addiction prior to offending.

Catrina said: "The message was clear and complex at the same time. Women are victims first before becoming offenders. You can see how domestic violence, poverty, addiction and lack of support can lead to prison. Society has failed these women and their families. We also found that women in prison or on probation can be funny and strong and intelligent, but that they can become trapped by the revolving door. Without societal change, an end to domestic violence, poverty and discrimination, you feared they would end up back in prison."

Open Clasp still works with the prison and the women incarcerated there, and continues to use theatre to fight for change. Catrina added: "Bringing women together with feminism at its heart can make change happen right in front of your eyes, and the plays created in response to all the magic that happens, the truth and reality, heart and rage, will actually change other people's worlds. It really is powerful, and we can open doors and help women's voices to fly high."

prison to get well

Believe it or not, some people look to prison for help. It's another issue that is difficult for those of us with relatively comfortable lives to comprehend. Why would anyone want to go to prison? But if you're experiencing major trauma in the home, or need help with drug use but can't access it in the community, prison might feel like your only option (again, it's down to limited choices).

This is something Beverley Hunter has come across a lot during her career. She said: "There were a lot of people coming in because they knew that in having their needs assessed they may be assigned a doctor or support team or drug worker they might feel unable to access in the community. They might get clean in prison or be prescribed a more manageable and legal substitute. But support in prison is a postcode lottery."

What Beverley means by this is that, while category D prisons (otherwise known as open prisons) are often geared up to provide holistic support for prisoners as they prepare for life back in the community, other categories of prison, including category B prisons where most prisoners go, do not always have that support. Beverley said: "There's research that shows that up to 70 per cent of people in prison have a mental health problem, but I think the reality is probably much higher."

In the United States, a 2014 article on the American Psychological Association website entitled 'Incarceration Nation' cites a National Research Council report. It says the research committee found that "the deinstitutionalization movement of the 1960s – which shut down large treatment facilities for the mentally ill – coupled with the lack of community resources to treat them, resulted in some people going to prisons and jails instead. One study found this trend accounts for about 7 per cent of prison population growth from 1980 to 2000, representing 40,000 to 72,000 people in prisons who would likely have been in mental hospitals in the past."

If this is a trend around the world, then clearly people are being punished for being unwell, or, as we've discovered, they are punished for being victims themselves. But inside prisons, there just isn't the resource to treat mental health problems either.

Beverley said: "When I worked for HMP Northumberland several years ago, we had 1,500 prisoners and only two CPNs (community psychiatric nurses). This meant that, as the majority of prisoners had mental health problems, they would often have to be supported by generalist healthcare workers. And for those with severe mental illness, if there was no space in the prison hospital, they might often find themselves in segregation for their own safety – something that is usually used to manage violent or disruptive prisoners."

mental health stigma in prison

Even if there is access to holistic and specialist addiction and mental health care in prison, are people willing and able to ask for it?

Beverley explained that, in male prisons especially, there is a significant stigma around mental health problems, especially among the younger population. She said: "If somebody was on self-harm or suicide watch, they were labelled by other prisoners as a victim or someone who couldn't cope inside. People don't want to be singled out like that. So many feel unable to ask for help for fear of being found out by other prisoners and bullied for it."

Beverley explained that there is also stigma among prison staff, due to their own nervousness around showing "weakness" or not being able to cope in the job, and that this can be transferred onto the prisoners. She said: "If you happen to be one of those prison officers who likes to help the prisoners, you might be labelled a do-gooder, as if it's a bad thing. So, when you've got the stigma within the prison community and the staff, combined with an increasingly low number of trained staff to support you, prison becomes a terribly detrimental place for those who struggle with mental health issues."

does stigma play a role in the sentences and support prisoners receive?

According to Richy Cunningham, the Ministry of Justice and the media play a significant role in the number of short sentences dished out for non-violent crimes. He said: "The 'tough on crime' message was something the Ministry of Justice would not move away from, no matter how much evidence we put forward on trauma-informed language and stigma. The media sends out messages that basically say that punishment – and only punishment – keeps the rest of the community safe – and that the more people we punish, the safer we all are (and the more likely you are to vote for the political party behind these media lines).

"It felt as though every decision made in the Ministry of Justice was given the 'tabloid test'. How might the tabloids twist the story and what might readers think of the current government – the fear of backlash for being too soft seemed to override common sense. For example, we've all seen comments on media articles about rehabilitation being 'fluffy' and a soft touch, perish the thought we should make life better for people who have committed an offence, to cope with their life. If an offender is helped back into their own accommodation to live a life free of addiction, how will the public view that? Will they be supportive of it? Probably, on the whole, not, because they see that there are others who are 'more deserving' of such support and in their eyes this is not the bloodthirsty punishment they crave for people they know very little about."

Richy explained to me that the media therefore focuses more on the tough actions taken – for example, a televised police documentary showing officers kicking the doors down to arrest dealers. He said: "It's always about the supply – rarely is the question of the need (demand) for drugs on the agenda. Why do people use drugs? Why do people need to emotionally escape their environment? Why do people find it easier to self-medicate through illicit drugs and alcohol to get their needs met more quickly? Throughout the, COVID pandemic, demand for drugs and alcohol increased, because some of our lives got worse. We were less connected and were suffering more pain both emotionally and physically due to fear, restrictions and inequality. COVID didn't create the demand for drugs and alcohol; it was us humans who wanted to change the way we felt, because we couldn't do anything else about the situation we were in. We could do well to show this level of understanding for people in the criminal justice system who didn't just have two years of a pandemic, but a life of trauma, deprivation, violence and shame from birth."

The problem with the "tough on crime" approach is that, while it might satisfy the public's appetite for punishment, it doesn't actually work. Beverley added: "There's so much research out there that proves that harsher and longer sentences don't work. But it's really hard to encourage spending on rehabilitative programmes by the kind of government that we have today when it's all about populism. The public want to see harsher sentences, so that's what they get."

This is another example of stigma influencing policy and funding, and therefore the services available to us. And this is why getting authentic stories with heart and emotion to the masses, like Open Clasp strives to do, is paramount. Because the public's empathy is minimal. Most of us are just too privileged to understand what others might have to go through. When our homes are safe, our educational attainment is good and our jobs are secure (or at least, our prospects half decent if we lose our job), we find it hard to really understand how it feels to live in poverty or with abuse or violence or trauma day by day. Living with a mental health problem when you have good support and safety around you is a different matter, so even for those of us with lived experience of mental ill health, sometimes we might find it difficult to understand why someone can't just see their doctor and enter treatment like we have. And so the public wants harsh sentences where prisoners are kept in basic cells with a mattress on the floor, a pot to piss in and three basic meals a day. But what impact will this have on prisoners?

"If you treat people like rubbish, like animals, they'll start to believe it," Beverley said. She is clear that the holiday camp perception of prison is nonsensical and that if prisoners have nothing to do – no purpose, no visits, no distractions – their wellbeing, and therefore their behaviours, will become more challenging. She said: "I remember when there was uproar about prisoners getting a TV. But when the TV sets came in, there was a palpable change overnight. It solved a lot of problems. Televisions aren't exactly giving people a luxurious life, and being glued to the telly isn't great for anyone, but at least it gave prisoners *some* form of activity, of focus. It's the same with young prisoners and games consoles. It's at least a form of activity that they can do."

It's interesting thinking about this in the context of the pandemic. Many of us have found lockdowns incredibly difficult, even though we are in our own homes, some of us lucky enough to live with family or much-loved pets. We have the freedom and means to speak to friends whenever we want, we can watch Netflix or Disney, listen to music, choose what we want to eat, move freely from room to room and go online whenever we like. But we still find it tough.

So, imagine what it's like if you have *no* choice or agency. And nothing to do. It's hardly a holiday camp allowing prisoners some down time to watch TV or play Mario Kart. Can anyone really believe that the best outcomes for prisoners and for society is if we leave prisoners to rot in a cell with nothing and no one? Would we rather pay for more and more indefinite sentences because the prison system makes people deteriorate rather than find hope and rehabilitation?

Some prison systems, however, take a different approach, as Beverley explained: "The Nordic model for prisons is really interesting. There's a high security prison in Norway where they treat their prisoners with respect and dignity, and offer lots of interventions to help with rehabilitation because they see them as a fellow citizen. Yes, they've fallen into bad ways or something's gone wrong in their life but they're still a part of the community. When they compared this to UK and US prisons the outcomes were very different. In the UK, for example, somebody might leave prison with £76 in their pocket and no follow-on support. So they end up back in exactly the same place where they started."

Interestingly, there is a stark difference in mental health spending in Norway compared to the United States. A special report by journalist Karen Bouffard for the *Detroit News*, who visited Halden prison in Norway, stated that, in 2013, 7 per cent of US health funding was spent on mental health, compared to 12 per cent in Norway. The article, part of an investigation to see how incarceration might be reduced in Michigan if it applied elements of Norway's practice, also stated that Michigan had an incarceration rate three times higher than Norway. The report says: "Critics argue that failings in the United States' mental health system have turned US jails and prisons into revolving doors for people with mental illness".

the impact

I spoke to people who had experience of the criminal justice system about the shame and stigma they have personally faced. Some felt unable to share even anonymous quotes because of the stigma attached to their experiences, and the individuals who have shared demonstrate why stigma is such a significant problem for so many people who have been in the prison system. Interestingly, both individuals who were happy to be quoted had significant mental health or drug problems prior to entering the system as well as experiences of trauma.

"I grew up in the care system and so didn't have the easiest childhood up by any stretch, but I do take responsibility for my choices and actions. However, I have experienced a lot of shame over the years because of this. When I was 16 I was arrested for possession of amphetamine. I remember the arresting officer telling me I was scum and that I'd spend many future years in jail. I ended up being involved in more crimes to fund my heroin addiction. Since being in prison, new girlfriends would Google me and find out I had this past and stop seeing me. I also lost out on a job because my DBS check came back showing the number of crimes I had been

involved with when I was using. Today I am eight years clean and sober, but shame and stigma really hinders that recovery. I'm just grateful I had Narcotics Anonymous to help me through it."

"My crime was trying to take my own life when I was in hospital. I was already seriously physically and mentally unwell having tried to poison myself. But because the way in which I tried to take my life risked harming others (I was in a single room when I tried to set fire to my bed, but because of the oxygen and things around me I later learned that the consequences could have been catastrophic), I was given a longer prison sentence. There was no intent to hurt anyone else and nobody did get hurt. Eventually, following my time in prison, I was moved into psychiatric care but the impact of the sentence has stayed with me."

"Because I came from a prison setting I was deemed 'undeserving' of treatment and felt bullied and intimidated by staff. I've even been accused of lying and making up that I had a mental illness just to get an easier deal in hospital."

It's clear from the topics already explored that stigma can impact on the policies, funding and therefore services available for mental health problems (particularly addiction). But when, for some people, particularly those with very challenging and chaotic upbringings and home lives, those problems lead to offending behaviours, there is further stigma.

The law says someone experienced a criminal offence therefore they are *bad* and they do not deserve support or rehabilitation.

Stigma goes in one end, and comes straight back out the other side, bigger and badder, and leaving those caught up in it stuck, disadvantaged, discriminated against and finding healthy living unsustainable if not impossible.

The recommendations in the Fulfilling Lives programme evaluation argue that "national sentencing guidelines must consider presumption against custodial sentences of less than six months for non-violent offences." That's issue number one tackled, but then what? How can people get help out of those situations that have led them to offend?

It's a much bigger problem than one that can be tackled in a book, but we are partly reducing stigma and discrimination if such recommendations come into force. At least it's one less piece of the shame and stigma jigsaw that people are forced to contend with. When individuals have multiple and complex disadvantages, surely as a society we shouldn't be so set on creating more problems for them?

Perhaps it's time to ask ourselves "Why?" before jumping to conclusions about anyone who's been in the criminal justice system. Perhaps it's time to reflect on our own privilege before condemning the actions of others. And perhaps it's time we stopped judging people according to their experience of an outdated, underfunded and stigmatized system.

With so many prisoners coming from experiences of domestic abuse and chaotic backgrounds, having undiagnosed developmental or mental health problems, or being desperate to escape the frightening world they live in by turning to drugs, it's not that hard to see that their behaviour is more a product of society's failings, rather than a product of their "badness".

12

"Asylums"

"What are you going as for Halloween?"
"A mental patient."

There are probably a gazillion Halloween costumes out there that play on the "mental patient" stereotype. A quick Google search will find brightly coloured T-shirts emblazoned with "PSYCH WARD OUTPATIENT" or "MENTAL ASYLUM INMATE". And if a T-shirt's not your thing you can go a step further and bag yourself a lovely Halloween straitjacket costume.

Yep, it's all *One Flew Over the Cuckoo's Nest* and creepy American teenage horror movies, isn't it?

It's night-time (psychiatric hospitals magically disappear in the daytime) *and through the dark and moody sky two torch lights appear to be getting closer. A sexy young couple come into view and approach the dilapidated old mental hospital. They break down the door overhung with ivy and spiders' webs, and they creak their way into the no-go zone of the entrance hall. Making their way down a corridor, bricks crumbling in front of their eyes, they pass what look like rusty instruments of torture hanging from hooks on cracked walls, before coming across an old, cold steel trolley complete with restraints. It's all too much for them – the fear, the excitement, the dirty old trolley (that they decide is a great place to get naked on) – and they immediately get to third base. The camera flashes on and off, and, between the glimpses of flesh we see a darkness ... There's something coming (and I don't just mean the couple) and when both of them (because it's the movies and it always happens at the same time) are simultaneously about to completely let loose with an orgasmic shriek of pure joy, a haunted mental patient slays them with his hooked arm. There's blood, there's screams, a chase ensues. Duh! Duh! DUHHHHHHH!*

I've just made this scene up – but we've all seen its type. I don't think I'm being a killjoy in saying that this tired old stereotype is more than ready for retirement. After all, when you've got poltergeists, demons and zombies to play with, you *really* don't need to toy with the old mental patient trope do you? I mean, you're not exactly going to be stuck for inspiration – there are enough scary things going on in the world.

Don't get me wrong, I've watched – and enjoyed – some of these movies in the past. And I've joined in with some pretty questionable Halloween fancy dress themes ("dead celebs" being one. I dressed as Nancy Spungen). But now I understand more about mental health, I feel that the mental patient horror theme is lazy. Because the idea of psychiatric inpatients being murderous demons or wretched freaks is based solely on a very, very old stereotype. And one that, in fact, only relates to mental illness in part ...

the history and the horror

Centuries ago, people would actually pay to enter psychiatric hospitals and see patients. Catharine Arnold, historian and author of *Bedlam: London and its Mad*, explained: "While there was definitely a voyeuristic element to this, it was also a fundraiser. Visitors to Bedlam hospital, along with other London hospitals, were asked to pay to come in and look around the hospital. A notice at the gates instructed: *Pray remember the poor LUNATICKS, and put your charity into the box with your own hands.*"

Catharine explained that, while some visitors were there for genuine reasons (i.e. the charitable giving), there was abuse. She said that in 1753 *The World* reported seeing a hundred people running riot during Easter Week. They were described as "making sport and diversion of the miserable inhabitants".

She added: "Conditions in these asylums ranged from above average – as in The Retreat at York, run by Quakers with humane and enlightened principles – to horrific, as in the case of York Asylum and, at times, Bedlam itself."

Bedlam Hospital was originally a religious order, run by the Church. Today it is a modern psychiatric facility known as Bethlem Royal Hospital and it is closely associated with

King's College, London and The Institute of Psychiatry, Psychology and Neuroscience. I know of people who have been treated there and who are grateful for the quality of support they received. So, we need to make very clear that, when we are talking of Bedlam, we are talking of the hospital in its former incarnation based on its former site(s) – many centuries ago. Something that we simply cannot compare to today's modern hospital.

But it is interesting to reflect on how the hospital that inspired so many horror movies was once run and how its name, which was contracted into "Bedlam", became a word to describe "uproar and confusion".

bedlam's patients

When I mentioned earlier that mental illness only accounted for part of Bedlam's history that's because the hospital was used to "deal with" people with a wide range of problems, including but not limited to mental ill health. It seems it was ultimately less about treatment and more about solving a "problem".

Catharine explained: "Bedlam took in anyone who fell under their broad classification of 'mad' – whether that be people with developmental problems, epilepsy, dementia, autism and conditions we might recognize today as Parkinson's or other nervous system diseases. Mental illness was of course included in this, with patients suffering from what we would now describe as schizophrenia or bipolar disorder also included. These patients were all lumped together and care was patchy, with well-documented instances of abuse and neglect by dishonest porters."

As Catharine put it, anyone considered "a bit different" would be swept into these dark, satanic institutions, and this even included unmarried mothers. Catharine also told me that patients could be admitted by their families who could not take care of them, and the poorest were admitted "on the parish", which meant that the church picked up the tab. She added: "For the poorest, it wasn't really about a cure. Many doctors were therapeutic pessimists who did not believe patients were capable of recovery. Classic treatments included 'leeching' (bleeding patients with live leeches), mustard plasters, cold baths and being strapped to a chair that whirled through the air like a fairground. There's certainly an argument that for the poorest, the asylums served as a catch-all to keep them off the street."

harmful stereotypes

Even though I am not a qualified, clinical professional, it's fairly safe to say that, all those years ago, patients will have probably seen any existing conditions worsen dramatically rather than improve. And you can probably say the same for the way treatments for physical illnesses were once carried out. A swig of whisky and biting down on a knife to prepare for limb amputation. Or perhaps you might have treated a bout of constipation with mercury?

But we see these physical treatments in history programmes and movies, so why can't we see the age-old asylums and straitjackets in movies? I guess the issue is that nobody really believes that if they went into hospital they'd be given a whisky and a knife to prep them for surgery but, believe it or not, many people *do* believe that psychiatric hospitals are all padded cells, straitjackets and maximum security cells with no windows. The harm? Well, if you had a mental health problem requiring hospitalization, and you thought you were going to a scary old padded cell in a straitjacket, you might not want to go. Thus problems get worse or anxiety and distress increases or, in some cases, someone is sectioned.

Additionally, we rarely hear about the other side of history – the more positive examples. Catharine told me about some of the better-run asylums helping people to learn a trade while on site receiving care, with some of the big asylums having farms, gardens and basket-weaving classes. And it's also interesting to remember that the definition of asylum is "a place of safety" – yet it's come to mean something completely different in the context of mental illness. It's become a stereotype. This is an example of how language changes and becomes problematic because of new associations we tag onto words.

Catharine added: "I can see why 'madness' would become a trope at Halloween – because we are frightened of what we cannot understand. So mental illness is consigned to the same category as the supernatural – ghosts, vampires, werewolves and zombies."

So, we need to all make an effort to understand mental illness and psychiatric care because, if we don't, it's harmful to the many people who experience it.

I know that these stereotypes still exist and have an impact on the public because, in 2019, I worked with colleagues on some research that evidenced it. St Andrew's Healthcare, a charity that manages a number of psychiatric hospitals, wanted to explore perceptions of modern-day psychiatric hospitals. The results were striking: 77 per cent of respondents indicated that they were fearful of being admitted to a psychiatric hospital, compared to just 31 per cent who were fearful of being admitted to a general hospital. Additionally, when presented with six images, around a third of respondents associated a psychiatric hospital with a padded cell. We also found that nervousness around those who had spent time in a psychiatric hospital, a prison or those who had been sectioned was higher in comparison to those who had self-harmed or attempted suicide.

What was more interesting was that those fearful of being admitted to a psychiatric hospital were significantly more likely to select the padded cell image.

I shared the same images with people who I knew had been admitted to a psychiatric hospital. Obviously, the sample was much smaller so this isn't statistically sound (it was a sample of 38 people) but, interestingly, not a single respondent selected the padded cell as being representative of a psychiatric hospital.

The stereotypes related to "asylums" and the people they treat also have an impact on the people who need to access inpatient psychiatric care today.

Mental health campaigner and author Jonny Benjamin was diagnosed with schizoaffective disorder and his symptoms have seen him admitted as an inpatient to various psychiatric hospitals over the years. He said: "It's very rare for people to ask if they can come and visit me while I'm in a psychiatric hospital. However, the one time I was admitted to a general hospital due to physical illness, I was inundated with requests from loved ones to see me."

Additionally, Dr Malkin of Harvard University has found that pretty much all of his patients have been nervous of inpatient psychiatric care. "Stereotypes definitely play a role here. Many people outside of mental health, who've never seen the inside of a psychiatric unit beyond dramatic portrayals through TV, movies or books, retain terrifying images; patients drooling on the electroshock therapy table, or staring vacantly into space or manically bouncing around a white room with rubber walls. As a result of these pervasive stereotypes, the idea of psychiatric hospitals literally terrifies patients, before I explain the reality to them."

This, along with the survey results, demonstrate that there is certainly still a fear – or at the very least a misunderstanding – about what inpatient psychiatric care is really like. Being in hospital is never going to be a fun time. But imagine if you've been admitted due to a mental illness, perhaps you've already experienced stigma relating to the illness itself. But now, when you're in unfamiliar surroundings, you're feeling even more alone because friends and family are too fearful or nervous about visiting.

the reality of inpatient psychiatric care

This chapter is certainly not trying to argue that all psychiatric hospitals or wards are nice, safe, comfortable places. Just like any health service – whether it be a general hospital, dental surgery, liver ward or maternal unit – there are good and bad examples. As Jonny told me: "My experiences of inpatient psychiatric care are very mixed. It is safe to say I have had more negative than positive experiences. However, for me, it is the care from staff that is always most valuable. Often, there are one or two nurses who I seem to connect with and who make a real difference to me. Thankfully, none of my stays as an in-patient have ever compared to those horror films!"

The horror films and TV shows that have depicted outdated or wholly inaccurate tropes include early films such as *Bedlam*, which starred Boris Karloff. Even though this film was released in the 1940s, Catharine Arnold says it was wildly inaccurate even for the time – never mind today. Other examples include films such as *One Flew Over the Cuckoo's Nest*, and, more recently, *American Horror Story: The Asylum*. You could argue that the latter ultimately tried to teach us that not everybody admitted to a psychiatric asylum was "crazy", but it also reinforced the "freak show" idea, as well as some of the terrifying treatments we might associate with the older horror movies. All in all, it was a stigmatizing and frightening depiction that anyone without prior experience of a psychiatric hospital might take as something close to reality.

But it couldn't be further from the truth.

Of course, we've also seen unsettling documentaries about psychiatric hospitals and they're based on fact, right? Well, yes, but that doesn't mean they are representative of psychiatric hospitals generally. You will often come across an investigative documentary that highlights poor patient care. That makes a programme – it gives the viewer a reason to tune in. It's about a scandal, about human rights. We find that interesting. When things are ticking along nicely, for example in a psychiatric ward where patient care is of a high standard, what's the angle for the programme? Will people tune in to a documentary with the headline "Journalist finds no cause for alarm at psychiatric hospital rated outstanding by the CQC?" Sadly, maintaining a quality service just doesn't draw in the audiences. So yes, the documentaries shine a light on the poorly performing hospitals, and that is a slice of the truth. But it is just one example out of many psychiatric hospitals.

Within psychiatric care there are so many different types of hospital or ward. For example, there are different levels of security – medium secure, low secure, etc.

– depending on how much of a risk somebody is deemed to be to themselves or others. You might also have single-sex or mixed-sex wards. In addition, there are specialist units, such as Mother and Baby Units (MBUs) that are designed to support women with severe postnatal mental illness. As the name suggests (and as I've discovered since working with the brilliant charity Action on Postpartum Psychosis), MBUs have more private, comfortable spaces for mums and their babies, and some even have facilities for partners to stay over. This is to ensure that mums are not separated from their baby at this critical time.

Additionally, some hospitals have pathways to independence, which might include onsite independent living skills and employability training facilities. St Andrew's Healthcare, I mentioned earlier, also has wards designed specifically for people with mental health problems who are also D/deaf or hard of hearing.

Of course, hospitals do still have a "safe room" (once called a padded cell), but these are very much there for the patient's benefit. Harvard psychologist, Dr Malkin explained: "These rooms will have a soft bed, soft furniture and a button to call for help. They're very much for the patient's benefit. With the exception of one extremely violent man we had on the unit who had to be retained and placed there, every single person I ever worked with as chief inpatient psychologist decided, in collaboration with myself and the wider team, that they would personally benefit from some time in the safe room."

the impact

I asked people who had experienced time in a psychiatric hospital what their experiences were like to get a more realistic understanding. I also asked how stigma has affected them. Here's what people shared with me:

"The first psychiatric ward I was admitted to when I was diagnosed with postpartum psychosis had a 'back entrance' which I think is because of the stigma that patients are subjected to when having psychiatric treatment. I'm not sure if it helped or made things worse, but I can see why the hospital felt it needed it. The second ward I was treated on was in some ways reminiscent of some of the buildings we might see in the movies – it was a big, old building and I remember it being really echoey with lots of long corridors with high ceilings. I didn't ever feel unsafe in there but, because it was a mixed sex ward, I wasn't especially comfortable either.

"However, I was transferred to a Mother and Baby Unit, which was completely different. Firstly, I was reunited with my baby, which made a huge difference to my recovery, but secondly, I had my own private space and it meant that my husband was able to visit."

"When I was first admitted to a psychiatric hospital, there was so much stigma around being sectioned and being 'mad' that I told people I was in prison instead, which I also had some experience of. It somehow seemed to conjure a less dangerous image and people responded better to that than to the truth. I think people I knew actually thought that I was

safer in a prison because of these ideas from the movies that I would be involuntarily medicated or locked in a padded cell. But it wasn't like that. In hospital I received holistic treatments – dialectical behavioural therapy, trauma therapy, meditation and mindfulness sessions. After many years in hospital I've had to dig hard to rehabilitate because of the stigma that still persists and I am still fearful of revealing the truth about my decade of inpatient treatment to new people. This is why today I try to speak openly about my experiences and take part in mental health campaigns. It's important to get the truth out there."

"I knew of the Bethlem hospital prior to being admitted. There are rumours that if you go into the basement rooms you can see where the shackles used to be attached to the walls, although I don't know how true that is. However, the Royal Bethlem Hospital today is actually stunning. I was admitted to the Mother and Baby Unit, where you have your own room and there are lots of lovely communal spaces, as well as spaces for arts activities and baby massage and occupational therapy. The grounds are beautiful too, there's an ancient woodland and wildflower meadows and these spaces were really important for my recovery."

---

changing perceptions

Dr Malkin says that education in schools is key. "There's no education about what actually takes place over the process for admission to a hospital. Inpatient psychiatric care shouldn't remain shrouded in mystery and fear. It needs to be brought out into the open more, to help people see it for what it is: another level of mental health care."

Of course, regardless of the standard of care received or types of treatments carried out in inpatient psychiatric wards, nobody wants to be admitted to hospital, and that's another area of stigma that persists. Some people believe that if they show even the slightest hint of suicidal ideation or of a psychotic episode that they will immediately be carted off under a section. But this isn't the case.

Dr Malkin said: "I tell everyone who suffers from intense distress that there's only one reason for hospitalization: a person poses an imminent threat to their own life or to others. And it has to be imminent – without supervision and care, they may kill themselves or someone else. That's a strict cut-off – and few people meet it. Most might have passing thoughts of death or odd ideas about their food being poisoned, or passive murderous fantasies that can be understood, managed and even eliminated. They might require ongoing assessment, but not necessarily inpatient care. Nearly all hospitalizations are collaborative – with the patient and clinician working together to determine, over time, if the work they're doing to heal and recover can safely be done outside a hospital. Inpatient care is for those who want and need it and the whole purpose of it is to maintain safety until they can continue their work outside of hospital."

Dr Malkin also told me about one patient he was working with who became so afraid of her suicidal fantasies that she could barely leave her room or work. When she finally decided she needed hospital care he spent time explaining the role of the hospital and walked with her, so she had somebody she trusted by her side when she was admitted. He added: "She felt good about her decision and was released within five days feeling much safer."

Dr Malkin added: "I often think of how many lives could be saved if everyone knew how psychiatric hospitalization really worked. All it requires is simple education."

Acknowledging that you need mental health support can be difficult enough given some of the stigma that still persists about various mental health problems. So overcoming that boundary and then being met with another – a fear of the very treatment you need to make you well again – makes the whole process exhausting and challenging. No mental health service is perfect, but we need to move past this idea that psychiatric hospitals are haunted houses with murderous doctors and freak show patients. And perhaps the reason we don't see many real-life examples on TV is because there isn't anything extraordinary about them. They are just hospitals treating patients, who want to get well.

conclusion

---

humanity first

Society today is far more polarized than anything I've ever experienced in my life. And because of this, we can often see people as with us or against us. But, as I've personally discovered, it's really important that we look beyond this diametrically opposed way of thinking and not see everything as either right or wrong.

Brexit, COVID, vaccinations, cancel culture ... the world sometimes feels like a hissing, spitting cauldron spewing out boiling hot animosity to anyone who dares to get too close.

Instead, I want to look at how I've used what I've learned and how I can continue to work on being aware of my biases and my own "lefty" echo chamber. It's so important to remember that there are human beings with fully fledged emotions sitting behind every tweet or Facebook post and even every news article that media platforms carry.

We'd all be much better off if we tried to step into someone else's shoes before firing shots of venom across our various social media platforms ... and I'm saying this as someone who's been on the receiving end *and* dished out my fair share of rash opinions over the years.

This book has been written because stigma can kill. It's as simple as that. But we also need to remember that, just because we believe that we are right, it doesn't give us the right to cruelly troll or intimidate people who we believe are wrong.

There's no definitive right or wrong way to deal with stigma, but I wanted to share some of the things I've picked up through taking part in conversations and debates. And I'm really not trying to preach – I've learned most of these things by getting them wrong myself!

1. consider your intent

Be honest about what are you trying to achieve in challenging this incident of stigma that you've happened across. Is it someone you don't like? Are you trying to sound clever? Do you simply love having an opinion? *Or* can you see a real and concerning impact that the stigma might have? If it's the latter, great, challenge it. But think carefully about how you go about it … (see point 4)

2. consider *their* intent

There's a saying: "Don't assume negative intent." Let's be honest, it's really difficult not to sometimes. If you're a regular on platforms such as Twitter you'll know just how hotheaded and angry the environment can be. But not everybody is out to cause a stir. Not everybody is there to troll. If somebody has slipped a mental health reference into a non-mental health conversation (e.g. I'm *so* OCD my bookshelves are immaculate) consider whether they *really* meant any harm? It's highly likely that they didn't mean to cause offence. So be careful how you tackle it – if at all.

On the other hand, where platforms are huge and the authors of such posts are renowned for belittling mental health problems for fun and to court controversy then, in that case, just go for it if you feel confident enough (be prepared for a backlash of Twitter hate though – believe me, I've endured it).

3. consider *who* they are

There are human beings behind most pieces of web content. Whether it comes from an organization or an individual. Even global organizations have individuals posting on their behalf. Plus, some organizations might actually be small, family-run businesses. I guess I'm just saying that if something is taken personally, or if a "brand" becomes defensive, remember there are people behind those accounts. Challenge without becoming aggressive. After all, aggression usually just creates more aggression and with that in mind, it's best to go back to point 1 and consider your intent.

With conversations about mental health, it's also worth considering if the person you are about to challenge may themselves be struggling with a mental health problem. If they are part of the online mental health community because of their lived experience, and they happen to disagree with your stance on stigma, don't dismiss their experience because you believe it to be wrong. Debate it for sure, but always be kind and respectful.

4. consider *how* you challenge

There's no hard or fast rule here. However, if you feel that something has been shared that could have a negative impact on people with mental health problems, but it has been shared by somebody who probably didn't mean any harm, think about challenging it discreetly. Send a direct message or email if you can. After all, this isn't about causing more shame; it's about having an open dialogue and sharing experiences. If you do decide to challenge publicly, just be thoughtful about how you do it.

However, if you're dealing with a regular purveyor of stigma who clearly knows what they are doing and has millions of followers lapping up their every tweet, just go with your gut and spew it all out!

5. don't get personal

OK so I might be guilty of this one, unable to contain my Twitter rants about various right-wing divisive figures, only to be hurled with insults from their loyal supporters. I learned two things here. Firstly, insults are pointless. I shouldn't have insulted – I should have called out what they were doing – not who they were. But also, the response I received was in no way relevant to the conversation. People commented on my face. I was lucky that the tweeter in question said I had a "square chin" because I spent years being paranoid about having no chin – so it was an accidentally welcome insult that had the opposite effect. But that was just a fluke. If they'd called me chinless it would have probably set me back years!

Never get personal – facial features don't determine words and values after all.

other things we can do

There is no definitive right or wrong way to challenge stigma, but, as discussed with Dr Ihemere in Chapter 1 (see page 14), language *is* powerful and its power can cause distress. You don't need to be an avid online stigma-buster who blogs about every mental health stereotype on TV to play an important role in tackling shame and discrimination. I write a lot about mental health because I have experienced a mental health problem, I've experienced stigma and I've read *a lot* on the subject. However, when it comes to race, I know I need to position myself differently and I have got this wrong in the past. I need to read more from experts, ask more questions and yes — call out racism. But I still have so much to learn because I have never been discriminated against because of my skin colour. So, learning and reading and trying to understand is really important.

With that in mind, turn to the back of the book where I've listed some useful resources and books that I wholeheartedly recommend to understand more about mental health more generally.

Taking a look at Natasha Devon's Mental Health Media Charter and the media guidance on both the Mind and Samaritan's websites are also key.

there is no "type" of person with a mental health problem

I'd like to finish on something about humanity that is really important to me. There is no *type* of person who experiences a mental health problem. Mental health problems aren't intrinsically linked to our personalities.

As Natasha Devon says, we're not here to say that you should like everyone with a mental health problem – mental health problems don't discriminate. So yes, some people with mental health problems will, naturally, be arseholes. And that's subjective too. I reckon there are enough people out there who think I'm an arsehole – but I have some lovely friends too (three cats and a long-suffering husband for starters).

A few years ago, I wrote an article for Sarah Millican's *Standard Issue* magazine called "A Series of Unfortunate Stereotypes". It was about how you can't judge somebody's personality based on their mental health problem. This became a fortnightly column called *It REALLY couldn't happen to a nicer* …

The idea was to put people into boxes relating to their job or personal tastes to show that, when it comes to mental ill health, none of these things matter. Mental health problems can affect those in positions of power, those with riches, those who are super-confident or seem like the life and soul of the party.

Here's a few examples.

- It REALLY couldn't happen to a nicer … Commando
- It REALLY couldn't happen to a nicer … Actor
- It REALLY couldn't happen to a nicer … Comedian
- It REALLY couldn't happen to a nicer … Teacher
- It REALLY couldn't happen to a nicer … Public Speaker

The point was, just because you struggle with anxiety, doesn't mean you're not going to be outgoing or strong. Or just because you are a highly disciplined army commando, doesn't mean you aren't going to experience problems with addiction.

Challenging mental health stigma and trying to learn more about how to have more positive conversations shouldn't be about sorting the woke from the chaff. It should be about learning from each other and sharing our knowledge and experiences. And we need to continue to learn *how* to do that because, if the 2020s so far have taught us anything, it's that life can very easily become divisive. The pandemic has become on a macro level what a family wedding is on a micro level – full of emotion and hot-headedness. Nobody's perfect in sparking the most considered and least judgemental conversation, but maybe we just need to give it a go.

As one in four of us will experience a mental health problem at some point in our lives, it's good to remember that mental health problems don't define us, and they don't discriminate. A lifelong friend is just as likely to be hit with depression as the school bully. The factors are diverse and often incomprehensible.

We don't have to like people because they are experiencing a mental health problem, but we shouldn't judge them on it either.

If there's one thing I've learned over the years, it's that nobody can argue with the following well-known idiom …

Don't judge a person until you've walked a mile in their shoes …

mental health helplines

UK
Mind – www.mind.org.uk
Samaritans – call 116 123

US
Mental Health America – www.mhnational.org
Crisis Text Line – text MHA to 741741

Australia
Mental Health Australia – www.mhaustralia.org
Lifeline – call 13 11 14

acknowledgements

Writing this book has been a huge team effort and I've been delighted to have the support and expertise of so many brilliant contributors who are all listed at the front of the book – Kaycey, Ruth, Natasha, Catharine, Jonny, Hope, Cara, Dot, Amy, Beverley, Maureen, Craig, Bernie, Shahroo, Helen, Stephanie, Luna, Adam, Claire, Jess, Richy and Catrina – as well as everyone who contacted me on social media to share their personal experiences. THANK YOU ALL. Your insights have been both fascinating and educational and I've enjoyed learning so much from you. A huge and special thank you goes to Sue Baker for her opening words and also her advice and support during the writing process. Sue, you have long been an inspiration to me and your work with Mind, Time to Change and Changing Minds Globally is something that has no doubt touched many millions of people around the world. Important and amazing work and I'm so proud that this book contains your words.

Thank you also to my fabulous and supportive editor, Beth; my publisher, Jo L for believing in me and encouraging the book; and of course my wonderfully patient agent Jo B who continues to smile through my over-excitability, always providing me with sound advice, support and virtual hugs every step of the way.

It goes without saying, but big love to my husband Chris and step-son Sam for encouraging me and tolerating my tenacious approach to writing.

references

FOREWORD: Time to change global (2022). *Conversations change lives: Global anti-stigma toolkit.* Available at: https://time-to-change.turtl. co/story/conversations-change-lives/page/1?teaser=yes (Accessed: 25 July 2022).

CHAPTER 1: Barton, L. (2014). 'Why not study Russell Brand for A-level English? Language evolves – get over it', *Guardian*, 7 May [Online]. Available at: https://www.theguardian.com/commentisfree/2014/ may/07/russell-brand-a-level-english-language-evolves (Accessed: 25 July 2022).

CHAPTER 2: Haslam-Ormerod, S. (2019). '"Snowflake millennial" label is inaccurate and reverses progress to destigmatise mental health', *The Conversation*, 11 January, [Online]. Available at: https://theconversation.com/snowflake-millennial-label-is-inaccurate-and-reverses-progress-to-destigmatise-mental-health-109667 (Accessed: 25 July 2022).

Powell, E. (2017). 'Piers Morgan slammed for "absolute ignorance" after claiming Will Young has "Whiny Needy Twerp Syndrome" not PTSD', *Evening Standard*, 30 May [Online]. Available at: https://www.standard.co.uk/showbiz/celebrity-news/ piers-morgan-slammed-for-absolute-ignorance-after-claiming-will-young-has-whiny-needy-twerp-syndrome-not-ptsd-a3552076.html (Accessed: 25 July 2022).

York, C. (2015). 'Katie Hopkins Depression Comments Call Some Suicidal People "Attention Seeking Bastards"', *Huffington Post*, 29 March [Online]. Available at: https://www.huffingtonpost.co.uk/2015/03/29/katie-hopkins-depression-twitter-_n_6964070.html (Accessed: 25 July 2022).

CHAPTER 3: BBC Radio 4 (2018). *Snowflake: from purity to overly-sensitive and easily-offended*, 27 October [Podcast]. Available at: https://www. bbc.co.uk/programmes/p06q967x (Accessed: 25 July 2022).

Brown, A. (2018). '46 Snowflake kids get lessons in chilling', *Daily Star*, 7 December 2018, Page 15.

The Week (2022). 'Where did the term snowflake come from?', *The Week*, 26 January [Online]. Available at: https:// www.theweek.co.uk/news/955539/where-did-the-term-snowflake-come-from (Accessed: 25 July 2022).

Fox, C. (2016). 'Why today's young women are just so FEEBLE: They can't cope with ANY ideas that challenge their right-on view of the world, says a top academic', *Daily Mail Online*, 9 June [Online]. Available at: https://www.dailymail.co.uk/femail/article-3632119/ Why-today-s-young-women-just-FEEBLE-t-cope-ideas-challenge-right-view-world-says-academic.html (Accessed: 25 July 2022).

REFERENCES

Morgan, P. (2019). 30 December [Twitter]. Available at: https://twitter.com/piersmorgan/status/1211667837670117378?lang=en-GB (Accessed: 25 July 2022).

TechnicallyRon. (2018). [Twitter] 7 March. Available at: https://twitter.com/technicallyron/status/971175455037513728?lang=en-GB (Accessed: 25 July 2022).

CHAPTER 4: Mental Health America (2022). *Depression.* Available at: https://www.mhanational.org/conditions/depression (Accessed: 25 July 2022).

CHAPTER 5: Mental Health Foundation (2022). *Mental health at work: statistics.* Available at: https://www.mentalhealth.org.uk/explore-mental-health/statistics/mental-health-work-statistics (Accessed: 25 July 2022).

Mental Health America (2022). *Mind the Workplace.* Alexandria, VA: Mental Health America. Available at: https://www.mhanational.org/mind-workplace (Accessed: 25 July 2022).

Duchaine, C., Aube, K. and Gilbert-Ouimet, M. et al (2020). 'Psychosocial Stressors at Work and the Risk of Sickness Absence Due to a Diagnosed Mental Disorder', JAMA Psychiatry, 77(8), pp. 842–851. Available at: https://jamanetwork.com/journals/jama-psychiatry/article-abstract/2763369 (Accessed: 25 July 2022).

Stansfeld, S. and Candy, B. (2006). 'Psychosocial work environment and mental health–a meta-analytic review', *JSTOR*, 32(6), pp. 443–462 [Online]. Available at: https://www.jstor.org/stable/40967597 (Accessed: 25 July 2022).

CHAPTER 6: Mind (2022). *What is psychosis?* Available at: https://www.mind.org.uk/information-support/types-of-mental-health-problems/psychosis/about-psychosis/ (Accessed: 25 July 2022).

Mental Health America (2022). *Schizophrenia.* Available at: https://www.mhanational.org/conditions/schizophrenia (Accessed: 25 July 2022).

World Health Organization (2022). *Schizophrenia.* Available at: https://www.who.int/news-room/fact-sheets/detail/schizophrenia (Accessed: 25 July 2022).

CHAPTER 7: NHS (2018). *Overview – Generalised anxiety disorder in adults.* Available at: https://www.nhs.uk/mental-health/conditions/generalised-anxiety-disorder/overview/ (Accessed: 25 July 2022).

MBRACE-UK (2021). *Saving Lives, Improving Mothers' Care: Lessons learned to inform maternity care from the UK and Ireland Confidential Enquiries into Maternal Deaths and Morbidity 2017-19.* MBRACE-UK. Available at: https://www.npeu.ox.ac.uk/assets/downloads/mbrrace-uk/reports/maternal-report-2021/MBRRACE-UK_Maternal_Report_2021_-_FINAL_-_WEB_VERSION.pdf (Accessed: 25 July 2022).

CHAPTER 8: Gage, S. (2021). *Say Why to Drugs: Everything You Need to Know About the Drugs We Take and Why We Get High.* Hodder & Stoughton

Office of the Surgeon General. (2020). *Facing Addiction in America: The Surgeon General's Spotlight on Opioids.* Independently published.

Walker, A. (2019). *Report reveals sever lack of services for UK opioid painkiller addicts.* Available at: https://www.theguardian.com/society/2019/nov/02/report-reveals-severe-lack-of-services-for-uk-opioid-painkiller-addicts (Accessed: 25 July 2022).

CHAPTER 9: Beat (2022). *Statistics for Journalists.* Available at: https://www.beateatingdisorders.org.uk/media-centre/eating-disorder-statistics/ (Accessed: 25 July 2022).

National Eating Disorders Collaboration (2022). *Eating Disorders in Australia.* Available at: https://nedc.com.au/eating-disorders/eating-disorders-explained/the-facts/eating-disorders-in-australia/ (Accessed: 25 July 2022).

Mental Health America (2022). *Eating Disorders.* Available at: https://mhanational.org/conditions/eating-disorders (Accessed: 25 July 2022).

CHAPTER 10: Mind. (2022). *About BPD.* Available at: https://www.mind.org.uk/information-support/types-of-mental-health-problems/borderline-personality-disorder-bpd/about-bpd/ (Accessed: 25 July 2022).

CHAPTER 11: CFE Research and The University of Sheffield, with the Systems Change Action Network (2020). 'Supporting people with multiple needs.' Available at: https://www.tnlcommunityfund.org.uk/media/insights/documents/Report-Summary-Improving-access-to-mental-health-support-for-people-experiencing-multiple-disadvantage-January-2020.pdf?mtime=20200316152718&focal=none (Accessed: 25 July 2022).

American Psychological Association (2014). 'Incarceration nation', *American Psychological Association*, 45(9), p. 56 [Online]. Available at: https://www.apa.org/monitor/2014/10/incarceration (Accessed: 25 July 2022).

Bouffard, K. (2019). 'Could Norway's mental health focus reduce incarceration in Michigan?', *The Detroit News* [Online]. Available at: https://eu.detroitnews.com/story/news/special-reports/2019/10/10/norway-prison-model-fixing-mental-illness-problems-michigan-prisons/1504226001/#main-ContentSection (Accessed: 25 July 2022).

Fulfilling Lives Evaluation. (2021). *Why we need to invest in multiple disadvantage.* Available at: https://www.fulfillinglivesevaluation.org/wp-admin/admin-ajax.php?juwpfisadmin=false&action=wpfd&task=file.download&wpfd_category_id=324&wpfd_file_id=6928&token=07c220a222f97c-c65fd4fab01d0e05cc&preview=1 (Accessed: 25 July 2022).

further reading

General mental health and wellbeing

Benjamin, J. and Pflüger, B. (2021). *The Book of Hope: 101 Voices on Overcoming Adversity*. Bluebird Publishers.

Devon, N. (2018). *A Beginner's Guide to Being Mental: An A-Z*. Bluebird Publishers.

Izadi, S. (2021). *The Kindness Method*. Bluebird Publishers.

Anxiety

Eastham, C. (2021). *F**k, I think I'm Dying: How I Learned to Live With Panic*. Vintage Digital.

Eating Disorders

Lisette, C. (2022). *The Eating Disorder Recovery Journal*. Jessica Kingsley Publishers.

Virgo, H. (2019). *Stand Tall, Little Girl: Facing Up to Anorexia*. Trigger Publishing.

Addiction and recovery

Dresner, A. (2018). *My Fair Junkie: A Memoir of Getting Dirty and Staying Clean*. Hachette Books.

Experiences of Suicidal Ideation and Psychosis

Benjamin, J. and Pflüger, B. (2019). *The Stranger on the Bridge: My Journey from Suicidal Despair to Hope*. Bluebird.

Other specialist topics

Arnold, C. (2009). *Bedlam: London and its Mad*. Simon & Schuster UK.

Malkin, C. (2016). *Rethinking Narcissism: The Secret to Recognizing and Coping with Narcissists*. Harper Perennial.

Further reading about mental health stigma and media reporting

Natasha Devon (2017). *The Mental Health Media Charter*. Available at: https://www.natashadevon.com/the-mental-health-media-charter (Accessed: 25 July 2022).

Time to change (2022). *Global anti-stigma toolkit*. Available at: https://www.time-to-change.org.uk/about-us/what-we-did/our-global-work/global-anti-stigma-toolkit (Accessed: 25 July 2022).

About Us

Welbeck Balance publishes books dedicated to changing lives. Our mission is to deliver life-enhancing books to help improve your wellbeing so that you can live your life with greater clarity and meaning, wherever you are on life's journey. Our Trigger books are specifically devoted to opening up conversations about mental health and wellbeing.

Welbeck Balance and Trigger are part of the Welbeck Publishing Group – a globally recognized independent publisher. Welbeck are renowned for our innovative ideas, production values and developing long-lasting content. Our books have been translated into over 30 languages in more than 60 countries around the world.

If you love books, then join the club and sign up to our newsletter for exclusive offers, extracts, author interviews and more information.

www.welbeckpublishing.com   **www.triggerhub.org**

🐦 welbeckpublish   🐦 Triggercalm
📷 welbeckpublish   📷 Triggercalm
f welbeckuk   f Triggercalm

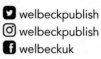

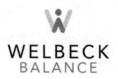

WELBECK
BALANCE

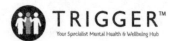

TRIGGER™
Your Specialist Mental Health & Wellbeing Hub